Atlas of Nuclear Medicine
Artifacts
and
Variants

Atlas of Nuclear Medicine Artifacts and Variants

U. Yun Ryo, M.D., Ph.D.

Division of Nuclear Medicine
Michael Reese Hospital
Associate Professor of Radiology & Medicine
Department of Radiology
University of Chicago
Pritzker School of Medicine
Chicago, Illinois

Carlos Bekerman, M.D.

Division of Nuclear Medicine
Michael Reese Hospital
Associate Professor of Radiology & Medicine
Department of Radiology
University of Chicago
Pritzker School of Medicine
Chicago, Illinois

Steven M. Pinsky, M.D.

Director, Division of Nuclear Medicine
Michael Reese Hospital
Associate Professor of Radiology & Medicine
Department of Radiology
University of Chicago
Pritzker School of Medicine
Chicago, Illinois

YEAR BOOK MEDICAL PUBLISHERS, INC.
CHICAGO

0 9 8 7 6 5 4 3 2 1

Library of Congress Cataloging in Publication Data

Ryo, U. Yun.
 Atlas of nuclear medicine artifacts and variants.

 Includes bibliographies and index.
 1. Radioisotope scanning—Atlases. 2. Diagnostic errors—Atlases. 3. Nuclear medicine—Atlases.
I. Bekerman, Carlos, 1939–   II. Pinsky, Steven.
III. Title. [DNLM: 1. Diagnostic Errors—atlases.
2. Radionuclide Imaging—atlases. WN 17 R995a]
RC78.7.R4R9 1985   616.07′57   84-19643
ISBN 0-8151-7489-6

Sponsoring editor: James D. Ryan
Editing supervisor: Frances M. Perveiler
Production project manager: Sharon W. Pepping
Proofroom supervisor: Shirley E. Taylor

To
Bann, Sue, and Other
Members of Our Families

Foreword

Primum no noxum (First, do no harm)! In therapeutic medicine this dictum is well known and generally appreciated. Its significance to nuclear medicine is, of course, do not diagnose what isn't there. Such misdiagnoses may sometimes lead to extensive efforts to fix what isn't broken, and, at best, much effort is usually expended to unwork the mischief.

This book was designed to prevent such diagnostic disasters as they relate to the practice of nuclear medicine. It is obviously an ongoing effort which will no doubt expand in future editions. I am particularly happy to see this work in print. "Artifact" and variant of normal should be the first category to be considered in every differential diagnosis of a nuclear medicine procedure. It also should be the first subject to be learned by starting residents. While the good teacher has a mental collection of such "lesions," he or she is often lacking in specific references or examples. Normal variants and artifacts have a way of not being adequately represented in the "teaching file." Some never get included because they are so "common." Others are excluded because of the physicians' embarrassment.

Dr. Ryo and his associates at Michael Reese have done a commendable job and a major service to the field of nuclear medicine. Hopefully, every new resident will carefully review this work and keep it available during the course of their training. It is also an excellent reference for even the most experienced of us. I suspect it will be used on many occasions to prove to a stubbornly unconvinced colleague that some "definite" abnormality is really nothing more than a figment of diagnostic imagination.

Paul B. Hoffer, M.D.
Professor of Diagnostic Radiology
Director, Section of Nuclear Medicine
Yale University
New Haven, Connecticut

Preface

THIS BOOK HAS BEEN DESIGNED to cover the field of nuclear medicine as the third in the series, Atlas of Normal Variants, the foundation of which was established by Dr. Theodore E. Keats. The recent publication of *Atlas of Computed Tomography Variants* has enhanced the roentgen variants series. We hope that this book will further enrich the series.

The 30-year history of multiorgan imaging in nuclear medicine is not comparable to the 80-year history of roentgen images. However, the experience with nuclear medicine images is extensive, and it is not too early to begin assembling variants and artifacts that may simulate a disease process on a radionuclide scan.

There is a basic difference between the radionuclide and roentgen images: radionuclide images demonstrate function, while the roentgen images represent structure. Moreover, the spatial resolution of radionuclide images is not exquisite enough to reveal details of anatomical variants in many systems. On the other hand, a physiologic variant may be accentuated on the functional images. Therefore, we encounter physiologic variants and artifacts that simulate disease process more frequently than we see anatomical variants. Fewer than half of cases contained in this book represent anatomical variants, the remainder are examples of physiologic variants or various artifacts that may mimic active disease.

We do not claim that this book contains all major variants and artifacts in nuclear medicine images. The illustrations from 320 patient cases shown probably represent only a fraction of such educational examples. However, we intended to show ways to recognize artifactitious lesions and variants.

We hope that this book will be helpful to physicians and technologists who are interested in radionuclide imaging. We look forward to receiving cases of proved normal variants from our readers. Such contributions will be included in future editions, with proper credits.

U. YUN RYO, M.D., PH.D.

CARLOS BEKERMAN, M.D.

STEVEN M. PINSKY, M.D.

Note: This book used radiopharmaceutical nomenclature recommended in the *Manual for Authors and Editors* of the American Medical Association. A large part of the nomenclature differs from that used by the *Journal of Nuclear Medicine* and by *Radiology*. Depending on the response of readers we may use the nomenclature as recommended by the *Journal of Nuclear Medicine* in future editions.

Contents

1
Technical Artifacts

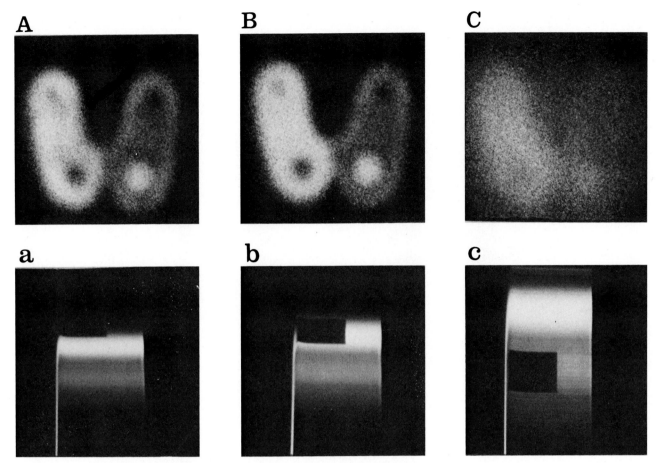

Case 1–1.—Instrumental Artifact in General; Improperly Set Photo-Peak

With a given gamma camera, resolution of the image is best when the photo-peak is properly set **(B and b).** A slightly deranged **(a)** or markedly deranged energy window **(c)** setting will result in a slightly **(A)** or markedly **(C)** deteriorated resolution of the image.

The photo-peak should be checked before every imaging procedure throughout the day.

Note b peak is slightly above the bar

OFF peak
Set on Xe¹³³

Case 1–2.—Technically Invalid Bone Image Obtained With Camera Window Set at Wrong Energy Peak; Instrumental Artifact

Posterior whole body bone image obtained using technetium Tc-99m medronate disodium on a 60-year-old woman shows overwhelming scatter photon activity and extremely poor resolution of the skeletal system **(A).** Window of the gamma camera was found to be set at photo-peak of 80 keV (for xenon Xe 133), thus recording mainly the scatter fraction of the Tc-99m photons.

The bone scan was immediately repeated using the proper photo-peak, showing excellent resolution of the skeletal system **(B).** Such poor resolution of the skeletal system **(A)** on a bone scan can be caused either by poor radiopharmaceutical quality or by poor instrumental control.

(Courtesy of William B. Martin, M.D., Division of Nuclear Medicine, Department of Radiology, University of Chicago Hospital, Chicago.).

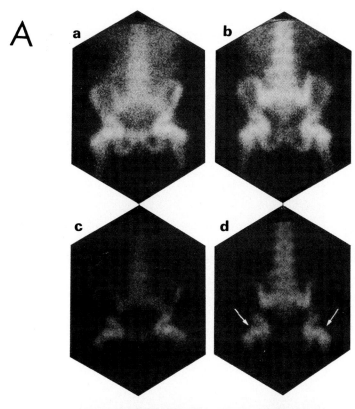

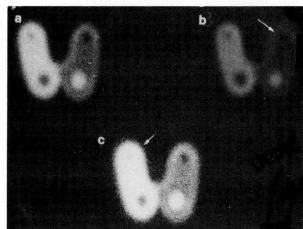

Case 1–3.—Instrumental Artifact; Importance of Optimum Intensity Setting

A, anterior **(a)** and posterior **(b)** pelvic bone images were obtained on a patient with bilateral hip joint active arthritis using technetium Tc-99m medronate disodium, and 300,000 counts were collected. Same views obtained collecting same 300,000 counts but with far lower intensity setting **(c** and **d).** Such underexposed scan images lose resolution of normal anatomical structures, particularly those with relatively lower radionuclide uptake.

Areas with increased uptake, "hot spots," however, may be demonstrated better on an underexposed image (**D,** *arrows*) than on a normally exposed image.

B, too high an intensity setting also causes deterioration of the resolution. A photopenic lesion in an organ with a high count rate will be lost on an overexposed image **(c),** while a photopenic lesion in a low count rate area will be lost on an underexposed image **(b).**

Again, a "hot" lesion is far less affected by improper adjustment of the intensity.

Intensity to high → low

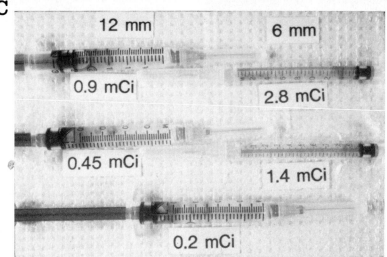

(handwritten annotations above image A) contain ↑ in activity Note ↑ in intensity + size   smaller syringe ↑ activity: Note intensity ↑ active in smaller volumes   opposite of A

Case 1–4.—Instrumental Artifact in General; Effect of Photon Flux on the Size of the Radionuclide Images

Radionuclide images of five syringes in two different sizes that contain various concentrations of sodium pertechnetate Tc-99m are obtained using a gamma camera with low-energy, parallel-hole collimator.

A, 1, 2, and **3** are images of same-sized (12-mm diameter) syringes but contain different concentrations of radioactivity—0.9, 0.45, and 0.2 mCi/ml, respectively. The higher the number of counts collected in a given intensity, the larger the image appears.

Images **4** and **5** represent syringes that are half the size (6-mm diameter) of syringes **1, 2,** or **3** but contain higher concentrations of the radionuclide.

B, images are from exactly the same objects as those in **A.** More numbers of counts are collected. Each syringe on the higher-count image appears to be larger than same syringe on the lower-count image. Higher count photon collections produce larger-looking images.

Comparison of the size of structures that have different radionuclide uptake rates on a scan may cause erroneous results. Evaluation of the size of bile ducts on a hepatobiliary scan, therefore, should be made with special caution.

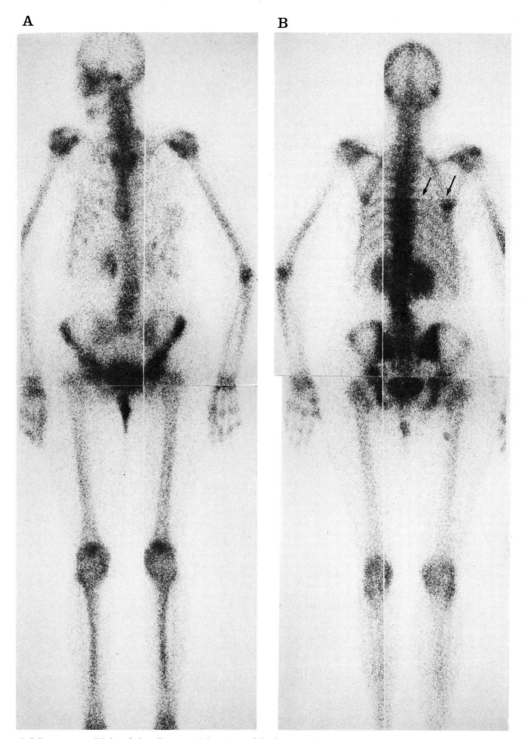

A **B**

Case 1–5.—A Momentary Halt of the Camera-Moving-table System Causing an Untoward Intensity Change on a Bone Scan; Instrumental Artifact

Anterior **(A)** and posterior **(B)** views of a whole body bone scan obtained using technetium Tc-99m medronate disodium on a 62-year-old woman with a history of right breast carcinoma shows no evidence of metastatic bone disease.

On the posterior image **(B)** there is sudden change of intensity *(arrows)*. The moving-table camera system was halted for a moment because the patient wished to cough. When the system was restarted, there was a change in the intensity. Such phenomena may occur due to unstable electrical voltage.

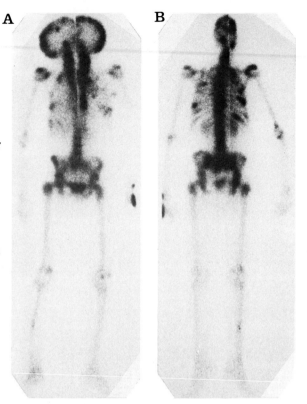

Case 1–6.—Double-headed and Microcephalic Figures on a Bone Scan; Positional Artifact

Anterior and posterior views of whole body bone scan obtained on a 56-year-old woman using technetium Tc-99m medronate disodium show a double-headed figure on the anterior image **(A).** The patient moved her upper body after the camera-moving-table made its first pass over the right side of her body, thus exposing almost her entire head on the first half of the bone scan, and exposing more than half of her chest and head on the second half of the bone imaging film.

On the posterior image **(B),** her head movement was the opposite that on the anterior image. Her head appears microcephalic because she moved her head after the camera made the first pass, removing the medial half of her posterior head from the imaging field.

A good technologist always explains the nature of the scanning procedure and emphasizes the importance of the position of the patient. Such communication will prevent motion artifact and also comfort the patient.

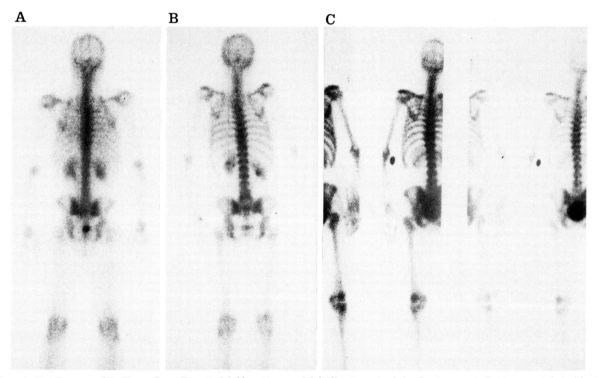

Case 1–7.—Poor-quality Bone Scan Due to Malfunction or Maladjustment of the Instrument; Instrumental Artifact

Posterior view bone scan obtained using technetium Tc-99m medronate disodium on a 47-year-old woman with breast carcinoma **(A)** shows poor resolution of the skeletal image with relatively high soft tissue activity. It was found that the energy window of the camera was accidentally set at 122 keV (Cobalt 57) instead of 140 keV (Tc-99m) at the time of the bone scan.

A posterior bone image obtained using the correct energy peak **(B)** shows a normal, good-quality bone image. An example of malfunction of an electrical circuit board in a gamma camera moving-table system is shown in **C.** Images of the second pass over the posterior right one-third of the body should be placed at the right side of the first image, with a minimum separation line ("zipper line"). In this case, however, the second image jumped to the left side of the first image, with infinitely wide zipper line due to an electrical circuit derangement. Such deranged whole body images may result from malpositioning of the detector orientation switch of the moving-table camera system.

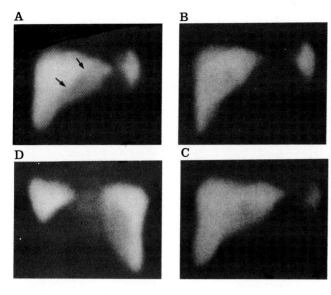

Case 1–8.—A Double-exposed Image on a Liver Scan; A Technical Artifact That May Cause a False Scan Interpretation

Liver and spleen scan was obtained using technetium Tc-99m sulfur colloid on a 57-year-old man with lung carcinoma.

An anterior view **(A)** showed diffusely decreased uptake in the lower half of the left lobe *(arrows),* initially thought to represent a gradual thinning of the left lobe. A left anterior oblique view **(B),** however, showed no evidence of unusual thinning or extrinsic compression of the left lobe.

A repeated anterior view **(C)** and a posterior view **(D)** were normal. The first anterior image **(A)** was a double-exposed image; anterior and left anterior oblique views. Such a technical error may cause a false scan interpretation.

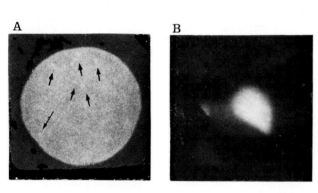

Case 1–9.—"Bad Crystal" of a Gamma Camera May Cause "Hot Spots" on a Scan; Example Case 1

A deteriorated sodium iodide crystal of a gamma camera can cause "hot" or "cold" artifactitious defects on a scan. The most common such detector artifacts are cold areas that may be corrected by readjustment of electrical gain of the photomultiplier tubes. When a crystal deterioration is severe, hot spots may appear on a flood field **(A)** and also on a scan **(B)** *(arrows).* An example shown here is a left anterior oblique view of a spleen with artifactitious hot spots.

"Crystal hydration" is proposed as a probable mechanism of such deterioration of the crystal by Nishiyama and his colleagues (*Radiology* 146:237, 1983).

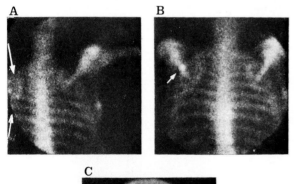

Case 1–10.—"Hot Spots" on a Bone Scan Caused by Poor Condition of the Detector Crystal of a Gamma Camera—Instrumental Artifact; Example Case 2

Posterior chest bone images obtained using technetium Tc-99m medronate disodium **(A and B)** show multiple small foci of increased uptake *(arrows).*

The location and number of the apparent lesions changed in each view. Flood field of the camera **(C)** shows numerous hot spots all over the field, another example of severely deteriorated crystal.

Such instrumental artifacts may cause false positive scan results when the scan is interpreted without reviewing the day's flood field.

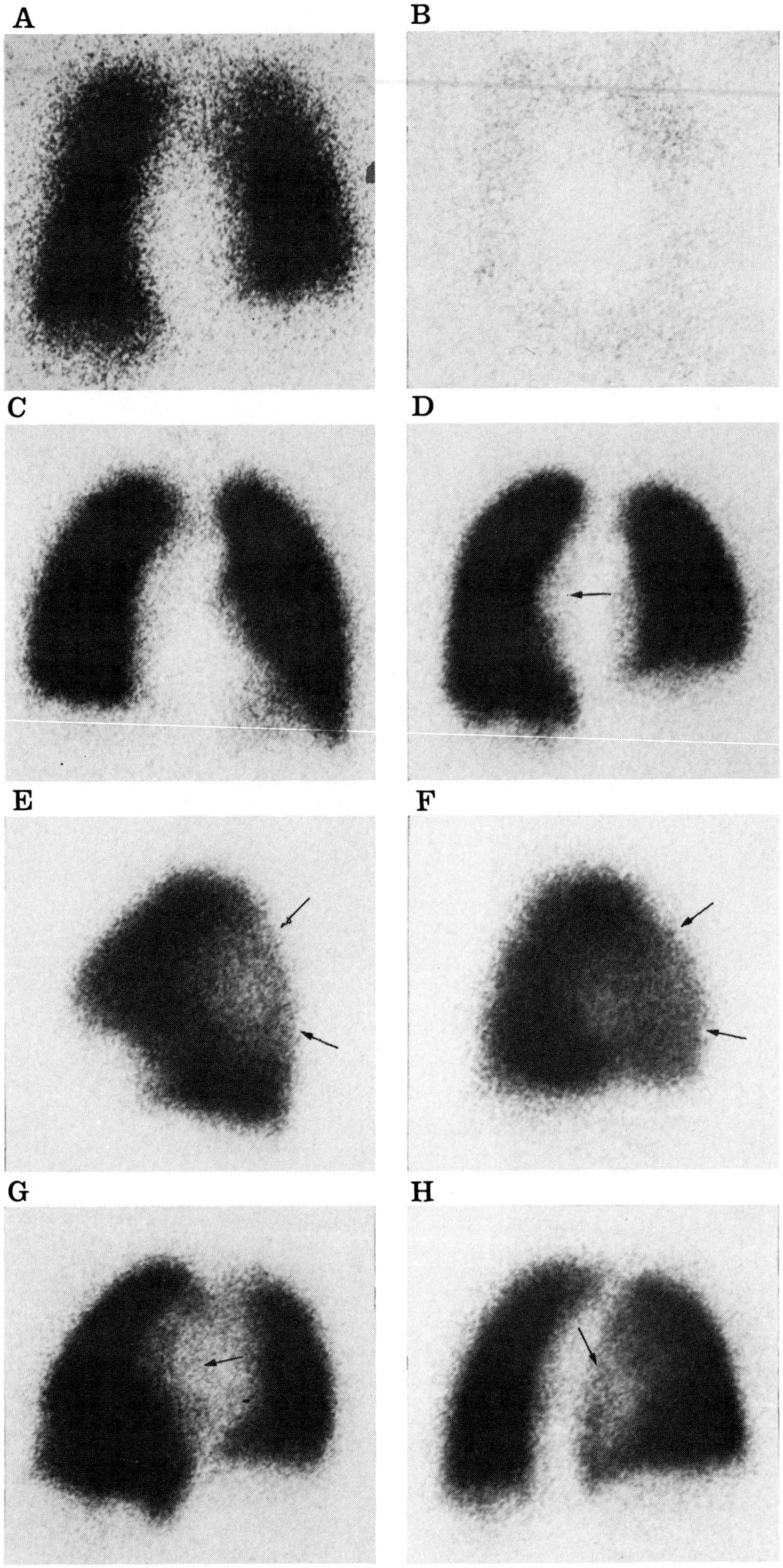

A

B

C

D

E

F

G

H

Case 1–11.—Perfusion Defects Caused by a Defective Photomultiplier Tube Demonstrated on a Lung Scan; Instrumental Artifact

Emergency ventilation-perfusion lung scan was performed using xenon Xe 133 and technetium Tc-99m macroaggregated albumin on a 49-year-old woman with chest pain and shortness of breath. Posterior view equilibrium and washout ventilation images (**A** and **B**) show an elevated right lung base and slightly widened mediastinum. The perfusion scan, anterior (**C**), posterior (**D**), left lateral (**E**), right lateral (**F**), left posterior oblique (**G**), and right posterior oblique (**H**) views, shows a large perfusion defect in the bilateral mid-lung fields *(arrows)*. The defects, however, appeared at different regions and were different sizes on each view *(arrows)*.

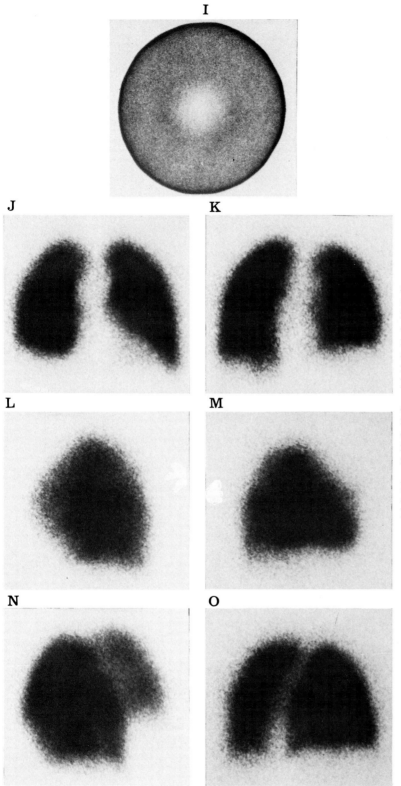

A flood field of the gamma camera taken after the lung study shows a large round defect in the center of the field (I), indicating that a photomultiplier tube in the center of the camera is not functioning. A repeated perfusion lung scan obtained using another gamma camera shows an elevated right lung base and otherwise normal perfusion distribution (J to O).

Comment: a radionuclide imaging should always follow the quality control of the instruments: photo-peak and flood field checks. These basic procedures are often ignored during weekend emergencies and may cause falsely positive study results.

(Courtesy of William B. Martin, M.D., Division of Nuclear Medicine, Department of Radiology, University of Chicago Hospital, Chicago.)

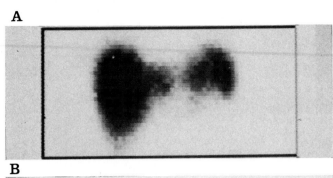

A

B

Case 1–12.—Instrumental Artifact; "Empty Liver and Spleen" Caused by Overflow on Emission Tomography of the Liver and Spleen; Example Case 1

Digital anterior view image of the liver and spleen **(A)** obtained using technetium Tc-99m sulfur colloid shows normal liver and slightly enlarged spleen.

Transaxial slices of emission tomograms of the liver and spleen, however, show diffusely decreased activity in the parenchyma of the liver and, in part, the spleen **(B** and **C,** *arrows*), creating images of "empty liver"; artifact caused by overflow of the recorder.

Areas with a number of counts higher than the maximum counts per picture element are burned out; thus, higher-count areas become empty on the image.

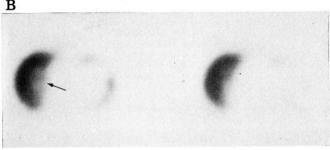

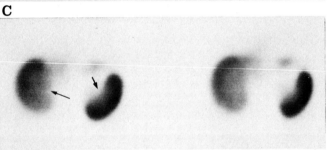

C

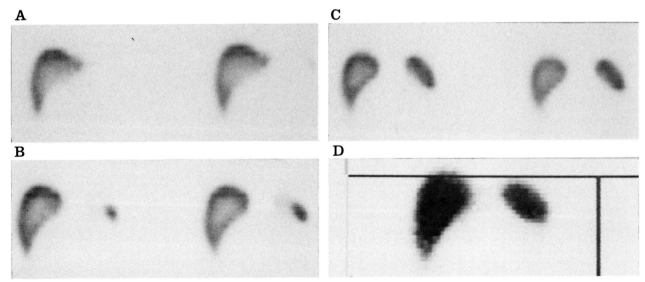

A

B

C

D

Case 1–13.—Instrumental Artifacts; "Empty Liver" on Emission Tomography, Example Case 2

Posterior digital image of the liver and spleen obtained using technetium Tc-99m sulfur colloid show normal liver and spleen **(D).**

Coronal slices of emission tomograms from anterior **(A)** to posterior **(C)** slices show empty liver; overflow image of the liver.

Such overflow images may be caused by a use of wrong collimator (high-sensitivity instead of high-resolution collimator), too high-dose an injection, or improper setting in sensitivity corrections.

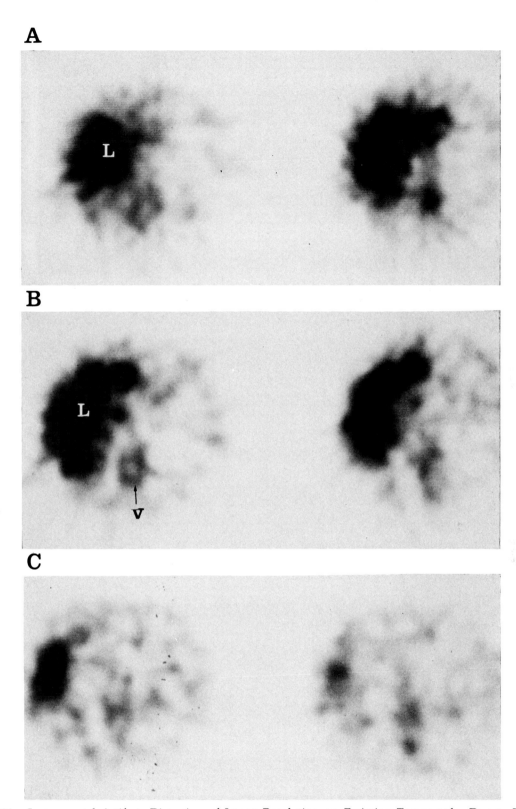

Case 1–14.—Instrumental Artifact; Distortion of Image Resolution on Emission Tomography Due to Lower Than Optimum Number of Counts

Transaxial slices of gallium citrate Ga 67 emission tomography of the abdomen, from upper **(A)** to lower quadrant **(C),** showing liver *(L)*, vertebrae *(V)*, and intestine. The images, however, are severely distorted, showing notably irregular borders of the organs. Such distortion of the resolution occurs on emission tomography when the counting rate is lower than optimum. The emission tomography thus might be less effective in evaluation of areas with low photon flux and in attempts to detect photopenic lesions.

2

The Brain

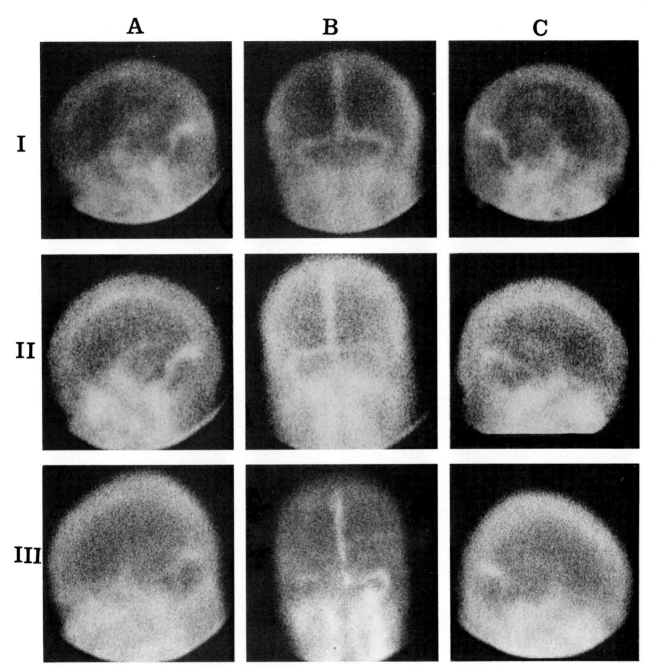

Case 2–1.—Transverse Sinuses of the Dura on a Brain Scan

Three example cases of the blood pool images of the brain obtained using an intravenous dose of technetium Tc-99m pentetic acid (DTPA) showing different pattern of the transverse sinuses.

The posterior **(B)**, left lateral **(A)**, and right lateral **(C)**, views of **case I** show an example of fairly symmetrical transverse sinus. **Case II** is an example of more prominent left transverse sinus. This form of asymmetry of the transverse sinus is the most uncommon among the three forms. **Case III** is the most frequently seen form, more prominent right transverse sinus.

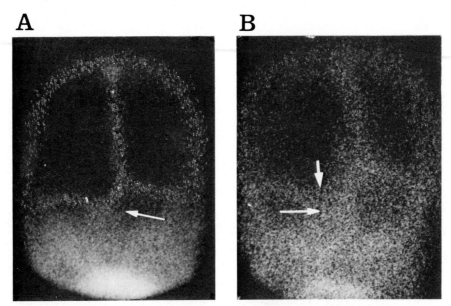

Case 2–2.—Prominent Occipital Sinus and Unusual Anastomoses With Transverse Sinus

Posterior view brain image obtained using sodium pertechnetate Tc-99m and a gamma camera with parallel-hole collimator **(A)** or with converging-hole collimator **(B)** show an unusually prominent occipital sinus *(long arrow)*.

The image of sinuses that are enlarged by use of the converging-hole collimator **(B)** shows the left transverse sinus anastomosed with the occipital sinus *(short arrow)*, a rare variant of drainage of the sinuses of the dura.

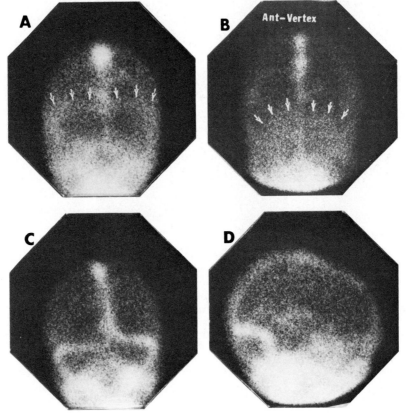

Case 2–3.—"Shine-through" Activity From Transverse Sinuses Seen on Anterior Blood Pool Images of the Brain

Anterior view **(A)** and anterovertex (chin-down) view **(B)** blood pool images of the brain obtained one minute after an intravenous injection of technetium Tc-99m pentetic acid show curvilinear **(A)** or diffuse **(B)** activity in the frontal region *(arrows)*.

Posterior **(C)** and right lateral views **(D)** show intense photon activity in the transverse sinuses corresponding to the activities (shine-through) seen on the anterior images.

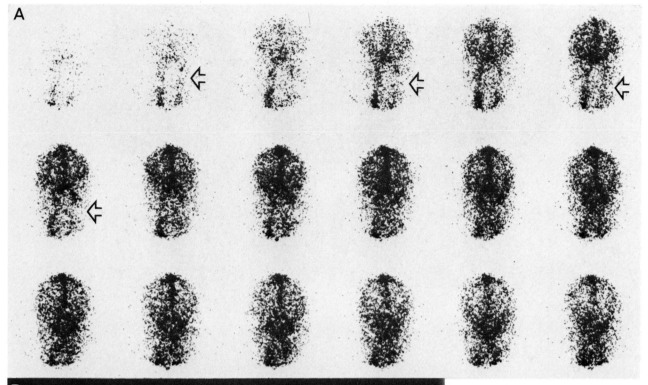

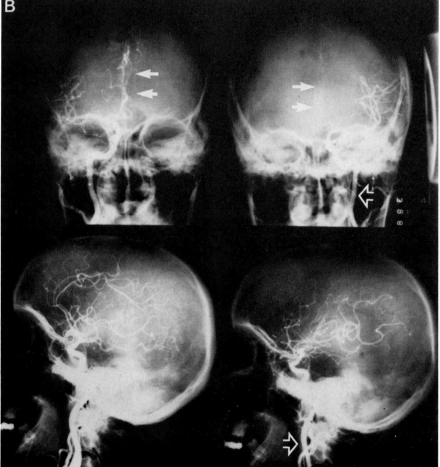

Case 2–4.—Asymmetry of the Internal Carotid Artery Causing False Positive Carotid Flow Images

A, dynamic flow images of the carotid arteries and brain on a 44-year-old man with seizure disorder. There is obvious flow interruption in the left carotid artery (*open arrow*).

B, the carotid angiogram showed asymmetry of the internal carotid artery, with the left side smaller (*open arrow*, 5-mm diameter, or 19.6 mm^2 cross-sectional area) than the right side (6-mm diameter, or 28.6 mm^2 area). The larger right internal carotid artery branched into the right middle and both anterior cerebral arteries (*solid arrows*), while the smaller left carotid artery branched only into the middle cerebral artery.

(Courtesy of Hussein M. Abdel-Dayem, M.D., Professor, Department of Radiology and Nuclear Medicine, Faculty of Medicine, Kuwait University, Safat, Kuwait, and George J. Alker, M.D., Director, Department of Diagnostic Imaging, Erie County Medical Center, Buffalo, N.Y.)

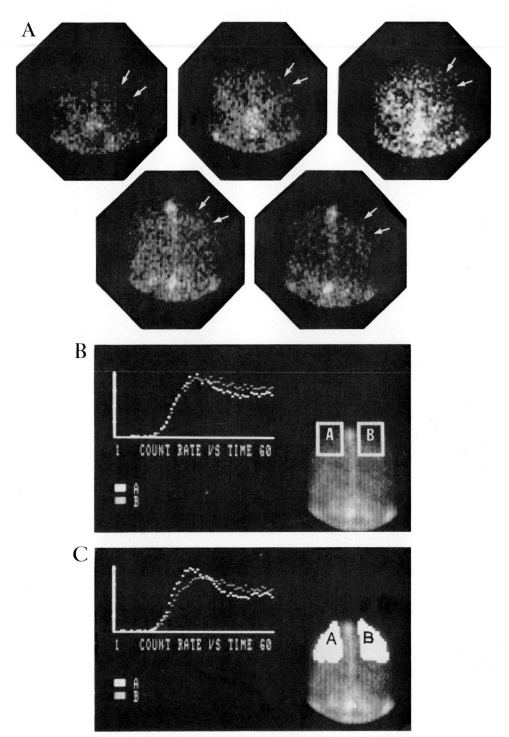

Case 2–5.—Time-Activity Curve of a Cerebral Flow Study Generated by a Computer May Cause False Study Results; An Example of Computer Artifact

A cerebral flow study, sequential flow images **(A)**, obtained using technetium Tc-99m pentetic acid on a patient with left subdural hematoma shows decreased arterial flow to the left hemisphere *(arrows)*.

A computer curve obtained from symmetrical, rectangular region of interest shows no difference in the slope of arterial flow in the both hemispheres **(B)**. Another computer analysis made using symmetrical but irregular regions of interest drawn along the hemisphere areas clearly demonstrates decreased arterial flow in the left hemisphere **(C)**.

The example case demonstrates crucial importance of selecting the region of interest in a computer data analysis. When a computer is used improperly, it may generate false results from any functional study.

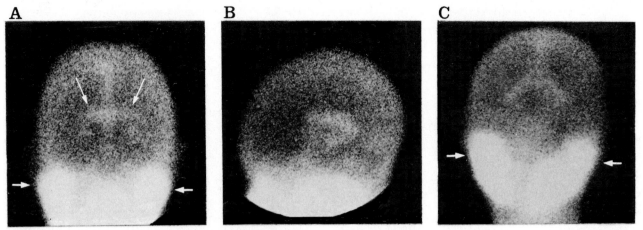

Case 2–6.—Images of Choroid Plexus on a Brain Scan

Anterior **(A)**, left lateral **(B)**, and posterior **(C)** images of the brain obtained 2½ hours after an injection of sodium pertechnetate Tc 99m show increased uptake in the lateral ventricles in the choroid plexus *(arrows)*. In addition, intense activity is seen in the parotid glands *(arrows)*. Such localization of sodium pertechnetate Tc 99m in the normal choroid plexus and the salivary gland is a common finding on a sodium pertechnetate Tc-99m brain scan when a patient is not pretreated with sodium perchlorate. (Potchen E.J., Mecready V.R. (eds.): *Progress in Nuclear Medicine,* Vol. 1. Baltimore, University Park Press, 1972, p 158.)

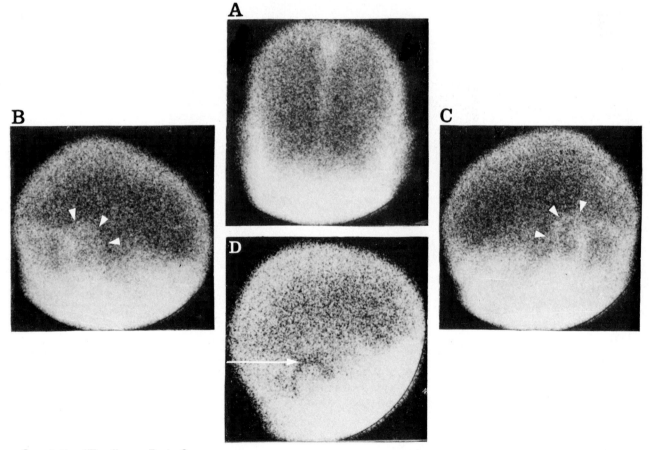

Case 2–7.—"Ears" on a Brain Scan

Anterior **(A)**, right lateral **(B)**, and left lateral view **(C)** brain scans obtained using technetium Tc-99m pentetic acid show round rim of increased uptake in the temporal region bilaterally *(arrowheads)*.

A lead marker placed along with helix of the right auricular **(D,** *arrow)* shows the rim activity on the lateral views to represent the auricular.

Visualization of the ear on a brain scan is a very common finding, though not routine. For a proper evaluation of the temporal region on a brain scan, it is recommended to tape the auricular down before the images are made.

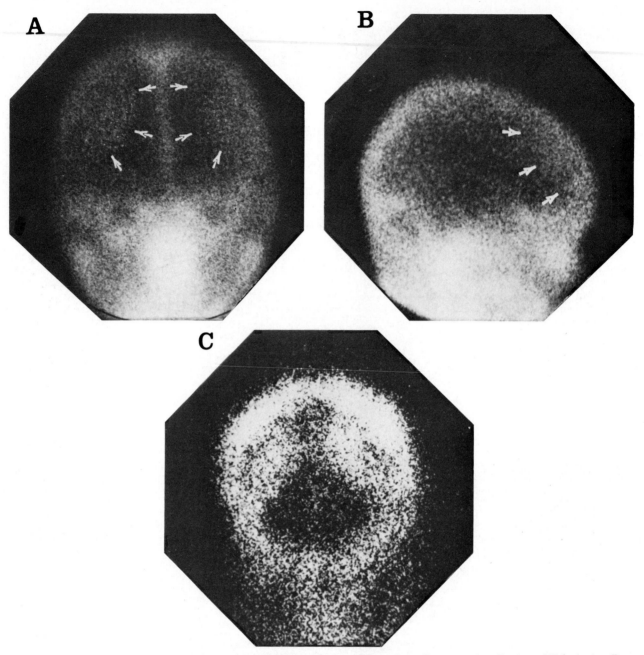

Case 2–8.—Increased Uptake in the Frontal-parietal Region on a Brain Scan Representing Regions With Active Bone Marrow Distribution

Anterior **(A)** and right lateral **(B)** views of a brain scan obtained two hours after an injection of technetium Tc-99m pentetic acid shows semilunar area of slightly increased uptake in the frontal-parietal region bilaterally.

Often, such bilateral frontal-parietal uptake represents distribution of active bone marrow in the skull as seen on a bone marrow scan obtained on the same patient using technetium Tc-99m mini-sulfur colloid **(C).** Areas of active bone marrow are more frequently seen on a brain scan obtained using sodium pertechnetate Tc-99m.

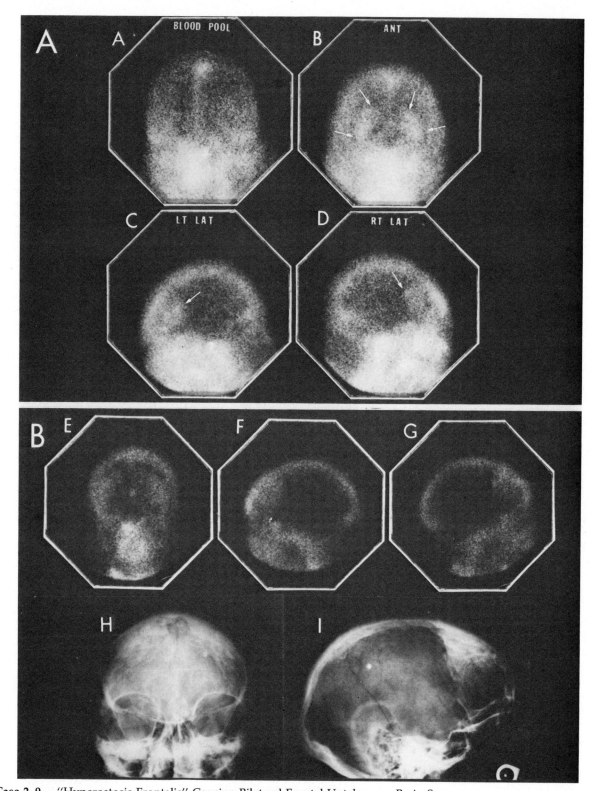

Case 2–9.—"Hyperostosis Frontalis" Causing Bilateral Frontal Uptake on a Brain Scan

Brain scan—anterior blood pool image **(A)**, delayed anterior **(B)**, left lateral **(C)**, and right lateral views **(D)**—obtained on a 38-year-old woman with headache, using technetium Tc-99m pentetic acid, shows abnormally increased intense uptake in the bilateral frontal region *(arrows)*.

The symmetrical, bifrontal lesion appears to be superficial on the lateral views, although the anterior view suggests probable lesions in the lateral ventricles or periventricular hemispheres. Bone scan of the skull—anterior **(E)**, left lateral **(F)**, right lateral **(G)** views—obtained on the same patient using technetium Tc-99m medronate disodium shows areas of increased bone uptake in the bilateral frontal skull, matching the brain scan findings.

Anterior **(H)** and right lateral **(I)** view skull radiographs show "hyperostosis frontalis," causing the abnormal uptake on the brain scan.

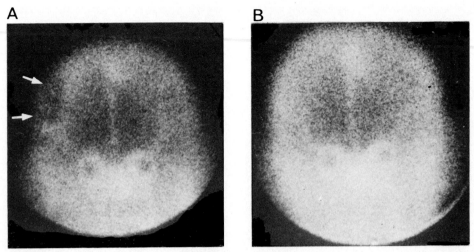

Case 2–10.—Attenuation Artifact Caused by a Nurse's Hand

Brain scan was obtained using technetium Tc-99m pentetic acid on a 65-year-old woman who had known lymphoma with probable intracranial spread. The anterior image **(A)** shows an irregular photon deficient area in the right parietal region *(arrows)*. The irregular defect corresponded to hand of a nurse who was holding the patient's head during the imaging. A repeated view after repositioning of the hand posteriorly **(B)** shows abnormally increased right subdural collection of the radioactivity.

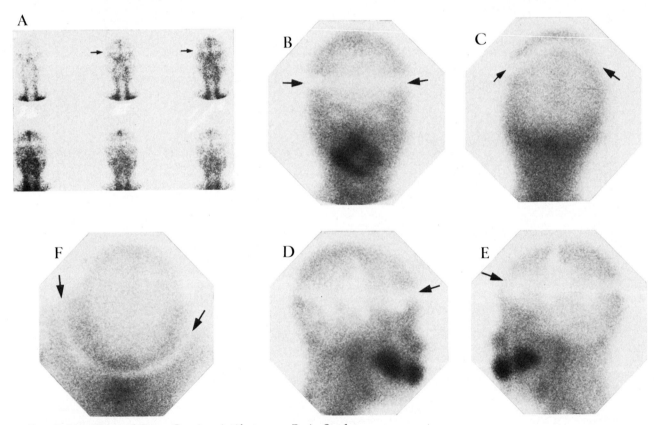

Case 2–11.—Cervical Brace Causing Artifacts on a Brain Study

A radionuclide cerebral flow study **(A)** and delayed brain scans were obtained on a 37-year-old man who was involved in an auto accident.

Cervical radiographs showed a fractured fifth cervical spine, therefore, a metal cervical brace was applied. A possible subdural hematoma was suspected because of severe headache. Computerized tomography, however, could not be performed because of the metallic brace. As an alternative procedure, cerebral flow study and brain scans were taken using sodium pertechnetate Tc-99m.

The flow images **(A)**, anterior **(B)**, posterior **(C)**, right **(D)** and left **(E)** lateral views and vertex **(F)** views, show band(s) of photon attenuation *(arrows)*. The attenuation line(s) appear over the hemispheres **(A,B,D,** and **E)** or outside the hemispheres **(C and F)**, thus indicating the brace that encircles the skull.

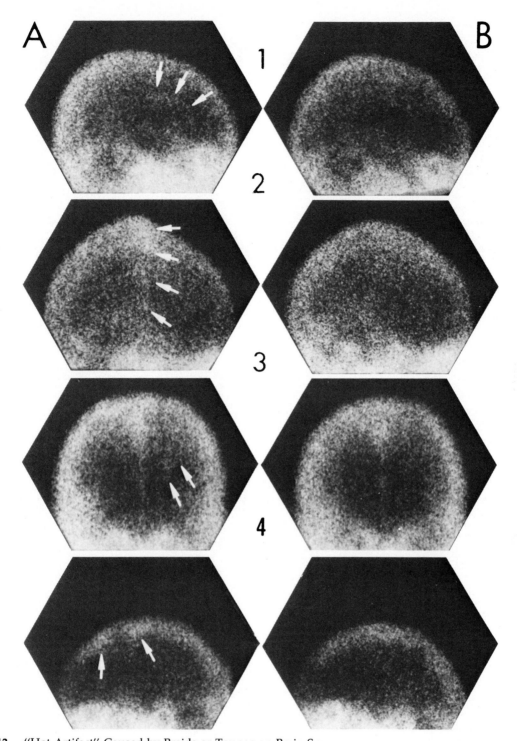

Case 2–12.—"Hot Artifact" Caused by Braids or Toupee on Brain Scan

Four example cases of brain images with various forms of "hot artifacts" caused by braids or toupee.

Cases 1 and 2: Right lateral view of brain scan shows crescent **(1)** or straight **(2)** band of accentuated activity (**A,** *arrows*). These patients had a short, thick braid tied over the right parietal region **(1)** or a long, thick braid **(2)** hanging over the right side of the head. These hot bands disappeared when repeated images were taken after the braids were loosened and combed **(B).**

Cases 3 and 4: Anterior **(3)** and left lateral **(4)** views of brain scan show irregular areas of slightly increased uptake (**A,** *arrows*). These areas corresponded to relatively thick toupees patients had over left frontal **(3)** or over left frontal-parietal areas **(4).** These areas of increased patchy uptake disappeared when the toupees were removed **(B).**

These hot artifacts on the brain scan represent bands of scattered photons (Ryo U.Y., Wilczak D.J., Kim I., et al.: Scan artifact caused by a band of scattered photons. *Radiology* 146:840, 1983.) Such scattered photons may lead to false positive brain scan interpretations on patients with thick braids or a toupee.

3
The Thyroid

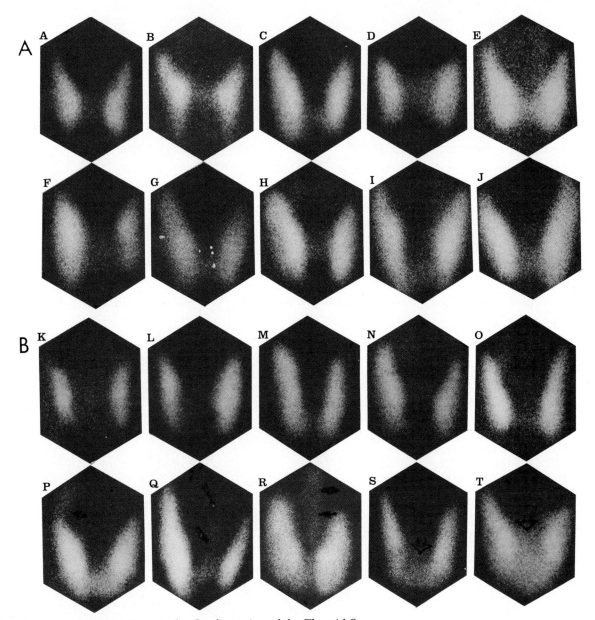

Case 3–1.—Normal Variations in the Configuration of the Thyroid Scan

There is wide variation in the configuration of "normal" thyroid on a scan. Image of a normal thyroid is not affected by difference in the imaging agent, sodium pertechnetate Tc-99m or sodium iodide I 123 (Ryo U.Y., Vaidya P.V., Schneider A.B., et al.: Thyroid imaging agents: A comparison of I 123 and Tc-99m pertechnetate. *Radiology* 148:819, 1983.); therefore, the agent used is not emphasized.

Ten examples of common variants and ten examples of less common variants, all obtained from euthyroid (normal) subjects, are shown:

A, typical, normal thyroid, symmetrical, small glands that become tapered at upper pole and round lower pole.

B, symmetrical, small glands, thinner at upper and lower pole.

C and **D,** small glands, slightly asymmetrical in size.

E, common, normal size and configuration, but lower poles almost fused together.

F to **H,** asymmetrical and not small (easily palpable) glands.

I and **J,** not enlarged, but tall glands.

K and **L,** small, atypical lobes, symmetrical **(K)** or asymmetrical **(L),** with wide separation of the lobes.

M, rod-shaped lobes, upper pole is not tapered, but round, as well as lower pole.

N, normal configuration of the lobes with tapering upper pole yet clearly asymmetrical in size; widely separated lobes without isthmus.

O, widely separated, tall lobes with faint visualization of the isthmus.

P, relatively thicker lobes, prominent isthmus, and functioning pyramidal lobe attached to the upper pole of the right lobe, a rare variant.

Q, markedly asymmetrical lobes with thin isthmus, and pyramidal lobe, a rare variant.

R, bilaterally thick lobes with clear visualization of pyramidal lobe. Usually such a scan finding suggests hyperthyroidism.

S and **T,** wide and thick isthmus or fused lobes with thin **(S)** or thick **(T)** lobes. Both are uncommon variants.

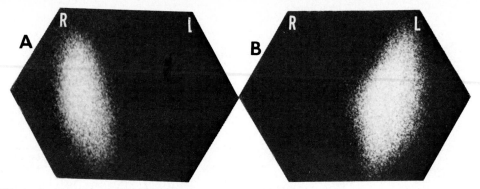

Case 3–2.—Hemiaplasia of the Thyroid Detected on a Thyroid Scan

Two example cases of unilateral agenesis of the thyroid. Thyroid scans were obtained using sodium iodide I 123 and a gamma camera attached with a pinhole collimator.

Case 1 (A) is a 25-year-old man with prior history of neck irradiation. His scan shows only the right lobe, which appears to be essentially normal. Neither the left lobe nor the isthmus is seen. Thyroid palpation revealed normal right lobe and nonpalpable left lobe. He had no history of surgery or thyroid disease, and thyroid function tests were all normal.

Case 2 (B) is a 27-year-old woman with childhood history of neck irradiation. Her scan shows only the left lobe, which appears to be slightly enlarged. The right lobe was neither imaged nor palpable. She had no history of thyroid surgery or disease.

Unilateral agenesis of the thyroid is a rare variant that is found in fewer than one in 1,000 of the population.

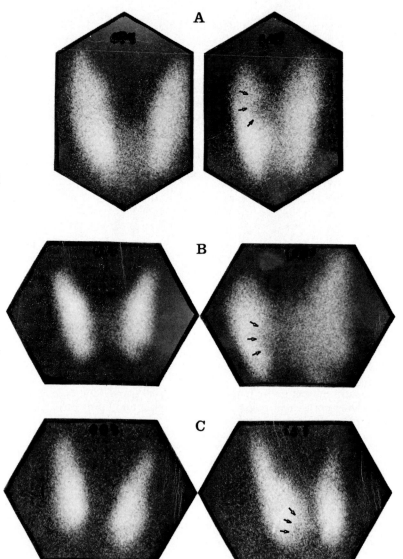

Case 3–3.—Artifactitious Lesions on Oblique View Thyroid Scan; Technical Artifact

Thyroid scans were obtained using sodium pertechnetate Tc-99m on three persons **(A to C)** with prior history of head and neck irradiation and normal thyroid palpation.

Anterior views **(left)** are all normal. Left anterior oblique views, however, show "cold" defect in the superior medial right lobe **(A)**, mid-medial right lobe **(B)**, and medial lower pole of the right lobe **(C)** *(arrows)*. These "lesions" are typical example cases of photon attenuation by adjacent structures, thyroid cartilage in **A** and **B**, and prominent sternoclavicular junction in **C**.

Because of such attenuation artifact, only the left lobe should be evaluated on a left oblique view and the right lobe only on a right oblique view of pinhole-thyroid images. (Ryo U.Y., Arnold J., Colman M. et al.: Thyroid scintigram. Sensitivity with sodium pertechnetate Tc-99m and gamma camera with pinhole collimator. *J.A.M.A.* 235:1235, 1976.)

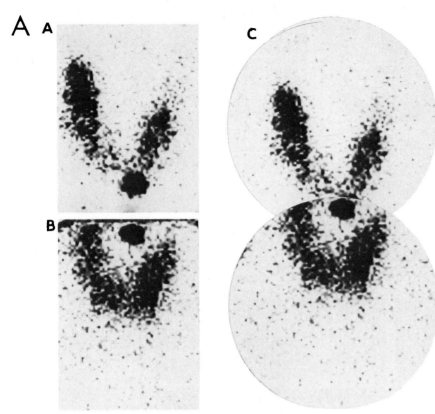

Case 3–4.—Double Thyroid? A Mirage on a Pinhole Scan

Artifact Caused by Spatial Distortion of the Pinhole Image. **A,** thyroid image obtained on a patient with suspected substernal thyroid **(a).** A hot marker was placed on the suprasternal notch, and the image was taken above the marker.

Second image **(b)** obtained below the marker, shows another thyroid below the sternal notch.

c, images of **a** and **b** were constructed and showed a double thyroid, one above and the other one below the sternal notch. This artifactitious double thyroid image was caused by the spatial distortion of the pinhole images. The mechanism is illustrated and formulated as shown in **B.**

(Courtesy of Michael A. King, Ph.D., and Lewis E. Braverman, M.D., University of Massachusetts Medical Center, Worcester, Mass. The mechanism was formulated by Ernest Byrom, Ph.D., Michael Reese Hospital and Medical Center, Chicago.)

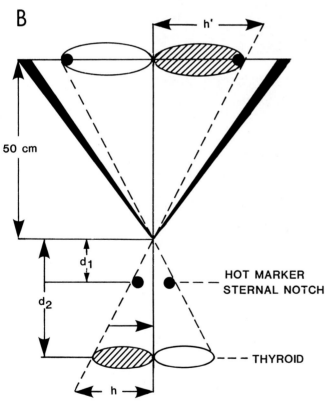

$h'/h = 50/d$

(1) MARKER AT DEPTH d_1

(2) THYROID AT DEPTH d_2

$h'_1 = 50h/d_1$, $h'_2 = 50h/d_2$

$\therefore d_1 = 50h/h'_1$, $d_2 = 50h/h'_2$

IF $h'_1 = 20$cm, then $h'_2 = 10$cm

$d_1 - d_2 = h50(1/20 - 1/10) = -2.5$ h cm

IF $h = 1$cm, then $d_1 - d_2 = 2.5$ cm

$d_2/d_1 = h'_1/h'_2 = 20/10$

∴ WHEN THE IMAGE OF THYROID MOVES 10CM ON THE FILM, THE IMAGE OF MARKER MOVES 20CM.

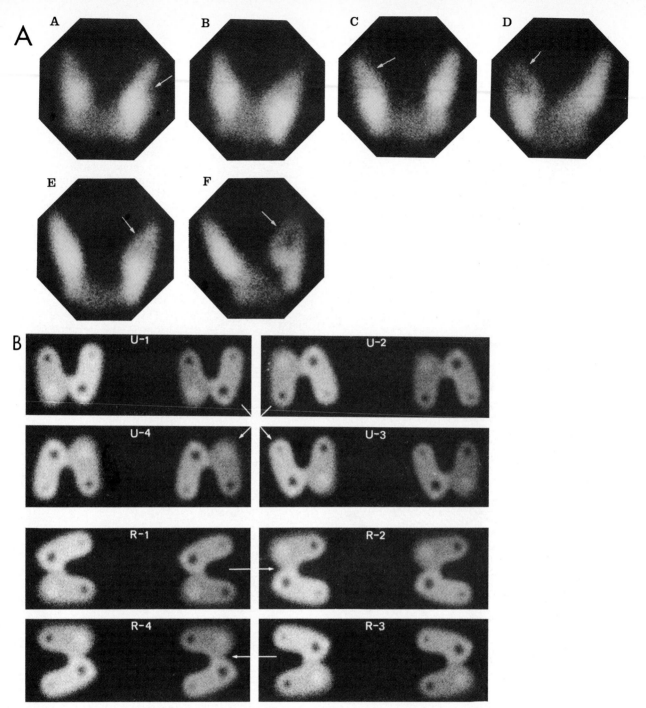

Case 3–5.—Cold Nodule in the Thyroid That Jumped From One Lobe to the Other on a Thyroid Scan; An Instrumental Artifact

A, thyroid scans, anterior and anterior oblique views, were obtained using sodium pertechnetate Tc-99m and a gamma camera attached with pinhole collimator on a 21-year-old man with prior history of head and neck irradiation. The first scan, anterior **(a)** and right anterior oblique **(b)** views taken in 1978, showed a cold lesion in the upper pole of the left lobe *(arrow)* that was not palpable. Follow-up scans, anterior **(c)** and left anterior oblique **(d)** views, were obtained four years later and showed a definite cold nodule in the right upper pole *(arrow)*. This time, however, a nodule was palpable in the left lobe.

Because of the discrepancy between physical findings and those on the scan, a repeated scan was taken a week later **(e and f)** and showed the cold nodule in the upper pole of the left lobe. This switch-over of the location of the cold nodule was caused by a wrong turn of the position switch of the gamma camera (Searle, Pho-Gamma IV). The camera has eight positional selections.

B, images of a thyroid phantom taken with the gamma camera and pinhole collimator at eight different position selections are shown:

U-1: Upright position 1; **U-2:** upright position 2; **U-3:** upright position 3; **U-4:** upright position 4; **R-1:** rotation position 1; **R-2:** rotation position 2; **R-3:** rotation position 3; **R-4:** rotation position 4.

On a thyroid scan it is not difficult to recognize a 90° or 180° rotation of an image. However, when the right and left side are switched, the rotation may not be recognized on the scan.

The switch-over occurs between **U-1** and **U-3**, **U-2** and **U-4**, **R-1** and **R-2**, and **R-3** and **R-4**.

Recent models of the gamma camera are known to be free of such positional pitfalls. However, when a thyroid scan is obtained using an older model of gamma camera and pinhole collimator, a given side of the patient's neck should be marked, using a radioactive marker, at the time of the scanning.

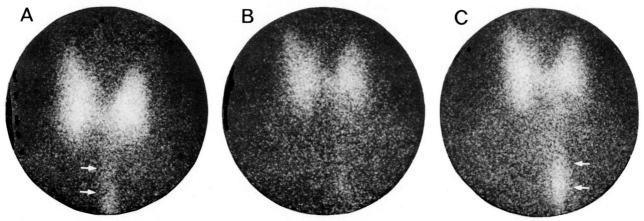

Case 3–6.—Sodium Pertechnetate Tc-99m Activity in the Esophagus on a Thyroid Scan

Routine, anterior-view thyroid scan obtained using sodium pertechnetate Tc-99m on a 26-year-old woman with a small (1-cm), soft nodule in the right lower thyroid shows a linear activity below the thyroid (**A**, *arrows*). The radionuclide activity in the esophagus is a common finding on a Tc-99m thyroid scan; therefore, a repeated image was taken after a couple of swallows of water (**B**). The localization of the radionuclide in the esophagus can also be confirmed by taking an image immediately after a swallow of small amount (less than 100 μCi) of the radionuclide (**C**).

(Comment: Differentiation of extrathyroidal localization of sodium pertechnetate Tc-99m from an esophageal activity is important because the former finding indicates probable metastatic thyroid carcinomas (Ryo U.Y., Stachura M.E., Schneider A.B., et al.: Significance of extrathyroidal uptake of Tc-99m and I-123 in the thyroid scan: Concise communication. *J. Nucl. Med.* 22:1039, 1981.)

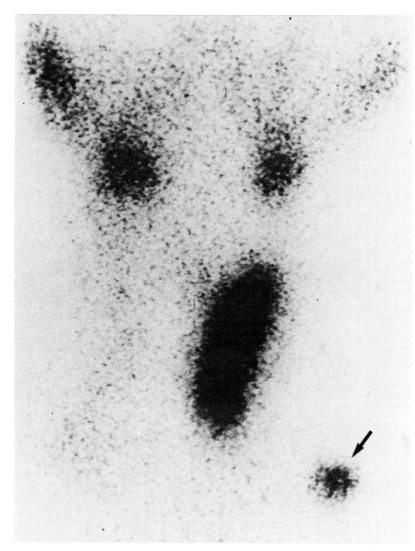

Case 3–7.—Vascular Retention of Sodium Pertechnetate Tc-99m Simulating Ectopic or Metastatic Thyroid Tissue

Thyroid scan obtained with sodium pertechnetate Tc-99m on a patient who underwent right lobectomy for a cold nodule showed a focal, extrathyroidal uptake in the left supraclavicular region *(arrow).* The abnormal focus of uptake simulated ectopic or metastatic thyroid tissue. However, the focus was later found to be a retention of the radionuclide in the left subclavian vein.

(Courtesy of Lopez O.L., Maisano E.R. [The Centro de Nuclear, San Miguel de Tucuman, Argentina]: Vascular retention of Tc-99m-pertechnetate simulating ectopic or metastatic thyroid tissue. *Clin. Nucl. Med.* 8:503, 1983.)

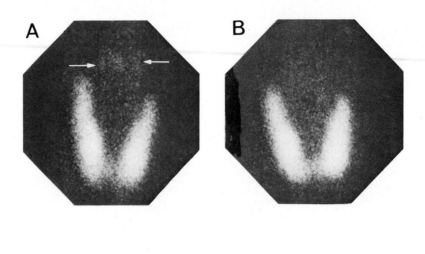

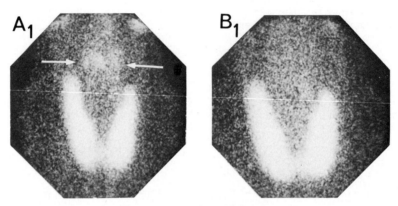

Case 3–8.—Radionuclide Retention in the Pharynx on a Thyroid Scan

Thyroid scan was obtained using sodium pertechnetate Tc-99m on a 39-year-old man with history of neck irradiation. Initial anterior images (normal **(A)** and high **(A1)** intensity) show irregular area of abnormal uptake in the midline upper neck *(arrows)*. This abnormal area of uptake disappeared on a repeated image taken after the patient drank a glass of water (normal **[B]** and high **[B1]** intensity).

Such unusual retention of radionuclide in the pharynx may cause false positive interpretation of Tc-99m-thyroid image as "extrathyroidal uptake."

Case 3–9.—Extrinsic Mass May Simulate Intrathyroidal Cold Nodule on a Thyroid Scan

Thyroid scan obtained using sodium pertechnetate Tc-99m **(A)** and later with sodium iodide I 123 **(B)** on a 39-year-old man with prior history of head and neck irradiation shows a large, cold nodule in the right lower pole *(arrow)*.

A firm, 2-cm nodule was palpable in the right lower thyroid on a physical examination. The nodule was surgically removed; it was a hyperplastic, extrathyroidal lymph node.

Extrinsic indentation of the thyroid by a lymph node or other mass cannot be easily differentiated on a scan from an intrathyroidal cold lesion.

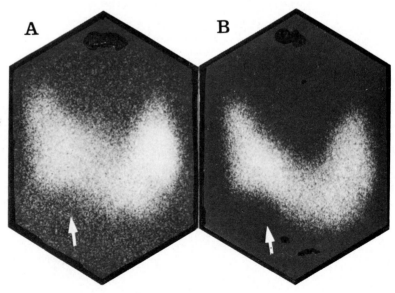

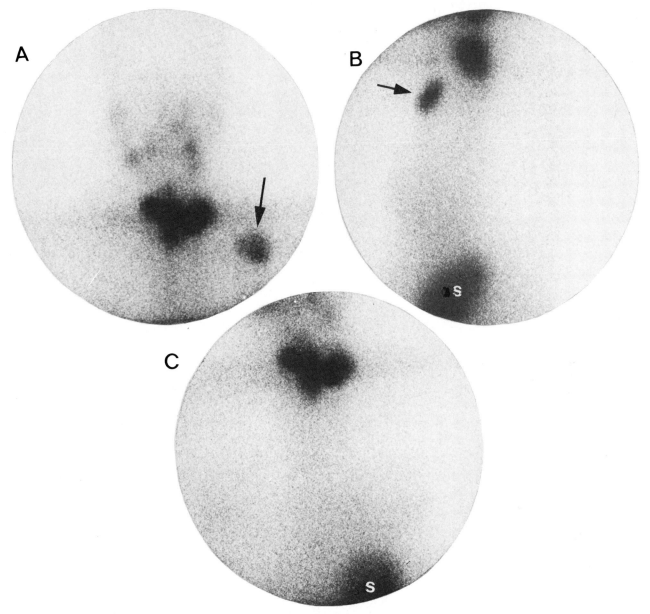

Case 3–10.—Metastatic Focus of Sodium Iodide I 131 on a Patient's Gown

Neck and chest scans were obtained 48 hours after an ablative dose of sodium iodide I 131, 100 mCi, on a 22-year-old man who underwent a near-total thyroidectomy for thyroid carcinoma with regional metastases.

Anterior neck and upper chest **(A)** view shows a focus of radioiodine uptake in the left upper chest *(arrow)* in addition to multiple metastatic foci in the neck region. Left lateral view **(B)** shows the abnormal uptake in the chest to be in the anterior chest wall *(arrow)*. However, the focal activity was contamination of the patient's gown by a drop of ^{131}I; the uptake disappeared on repeated chest view taken after the contaminated gown was changed (s = stomach).

4

The Lungs

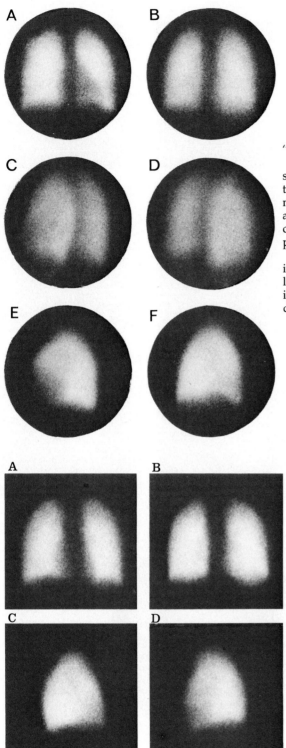

Case 4–1.—Normal Perfusion Lung Scan on a Patient With a "Small Heart"

Perfusion lung scan obtained on a 23-year-old woman with sudden onset of chest pain and shortness of breath using technetium Tc-99m macroaggregated albumin shows essentially normal distribution of the perfusion. The cardiac silhouette appears on the anterior view **(A)** as smaller than usual, and cardiac indentation in the left lower lobe is not apparent on the posterior image **(B).**

In the majority of perfusion lung scan cases, the cardiac indentation caused a large defect not only in the anterior left lung but also in the anterior base of the right middle lobe. But in this case with a small heart, cardiac indentation is not demonstrated on the right lateral image **(F).**

Case 4–2.—Invisible Cardiac Impression on a Perfusion Lung Scan

Perfusion lung scan, anterior **(A)**, posterior **(B)**, right lateral **(C)**, and left lateral **(D)** views, obtained on a 19-year-old girl with fractured left hip shows a normal distribution of the lung perfusion.

The normally prominent cardiac impression on the anterior and left lateral views is not obvious in this case because of the small heart; a rare variant seen on a perfusion lung scan.

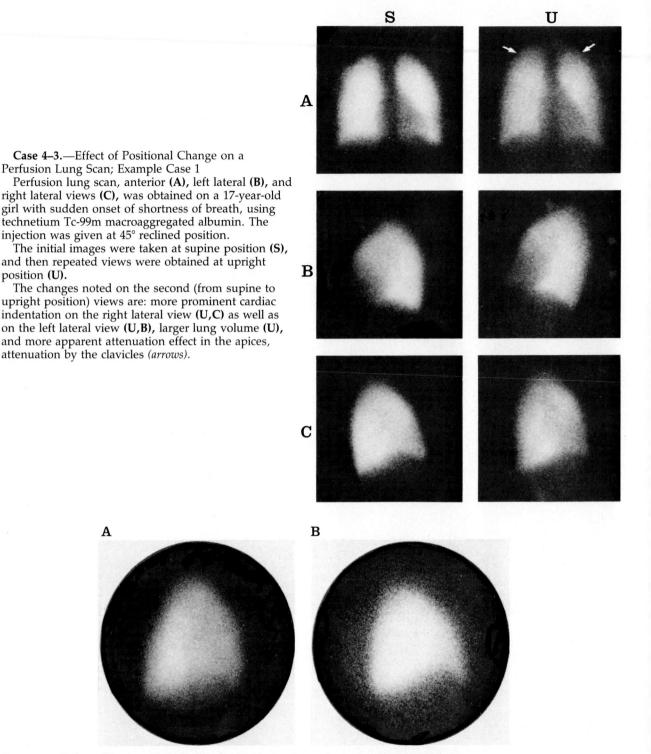

Case 4–3.—Effect of Positional Change on a Perfusion Lung Scan; Example Case 1

Perfusion lung scan, anterior **(A)**, left lateral **(B)**, and right lateral views **(C)**, was obtained on a 17-year-old girl with sudden onset of shortness of breath, using technetium Tc-99m macroaggregated albumin. The injection was given at 45° reclined position.

The initial images were taken at supine position **(S)**, and then repeated views were obtained at upright position **(U)**.

The changes noted on the second (from supine to upright position) views are: more prominent cardiac indentation on the right lateral view **(U,C)** as well as on the left lateral view **(U,B)**, larger lung volume **(U)**, and more apparent attenuation effect in the apices, attenuation by the clavicles *(arrows)*.

Case 4–4.—Effect of Positional Changes on a Perfusion Lung Scan; Example Case 2

Right lateral view perfusion lung image taken while the patient was in left decubitus position **(A)** shows diffusely decreased perfusion in the anterior half of the right lung.

A repeated view, same right lateral image, taken at upright position shows even distribution of the radioactivity **(B)**; another example that emphasizes the importance of the proper positioning of a patient to obtain a good-quality, valid radionuclide scan.

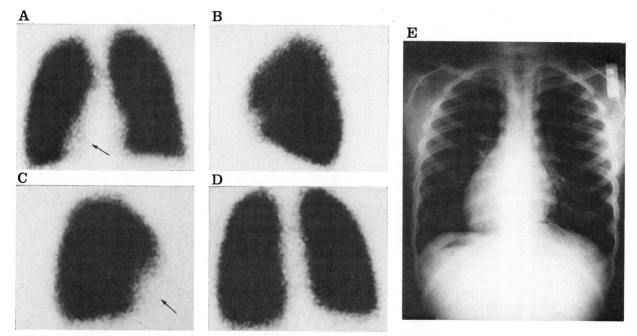

Case 4–5.—Kartagener's Syndrome; A Dextrocardia Detected on a Perfusion Lung Scan

Perfusion lung scan, anterior **(A)**, left lateral **(B)**, right lateral **(C)**, and posterior views **(D)**, obtained using technetium Tc-99m macroaggregated albumin on a 13-year-old boy with pneumonia, otitis, and sinusitis shows the cardiac impression in the right lung **(A** and **C,** *arrows*).

The left lateral view that normally shows the most prominent cardiac impression demonstrates only a minimal indentation **(B)**.

A chest radiograph of the patient **(E)** shows dextrocardia, one of the triad described in the rare hereditary disorder Kartagener's syndrome. (Bergstrom W.H., Cook C.D., Scannell J.G., et al.: Situs inversus, bronchiectasis and sinusitis. *Pediatrics* 6:573, 1950.)

(Courtesy of S. Sepahdari, M.D., Department of Radiology, Mercy Hospital and Medical Center, Chicago.)

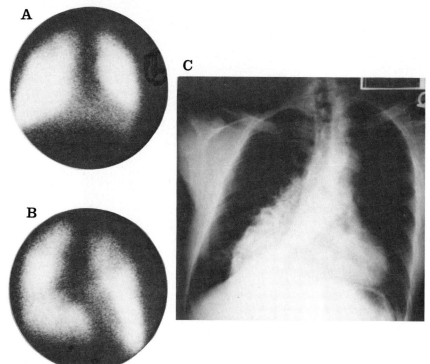

Case 4–6.—Deformation of the Lungs Due to Severe Scoliosis; Example Case 1

Anterior **(A)** and posterior **(B)** views of perfusion lung scan obtained using technetium Tc-99m macroaggregated albumin show markedly deformed architecture of the lungs with irregular distribution of the perfusion.

Such deformation of the lungs is a common consequence of severe scoliosis, as seen on a chest radiograph **(C)** of this case.

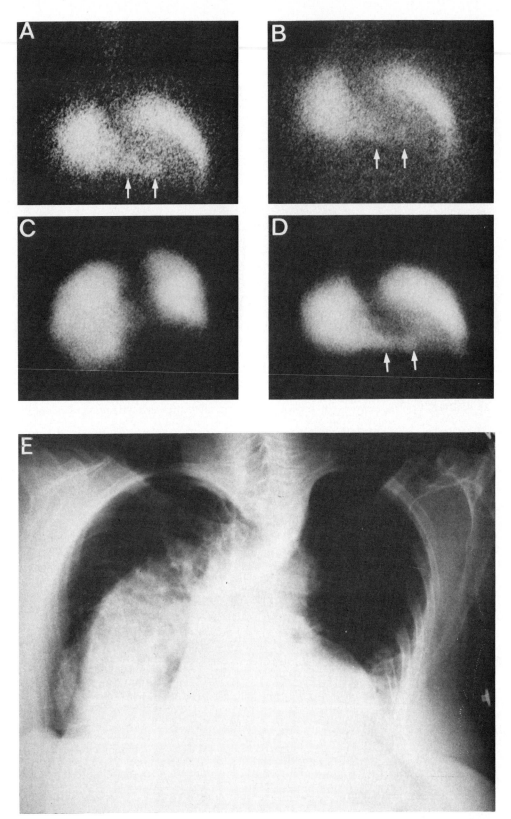

Case 4–7.—Anomalous Lungs Due to Severe Scoliosis; Example Case 2

Single-breath **(A)** and equilibrium **(B)** ventilation scan and anterior **(C)** and posterior **(D)** perfusion lung scan obtained on a 72-year-old woman with sudden onset of shortness of breath show a markedly distorted anatomy of the lungs, with herniation of the left lung into the right thorax *(arrows)*.

Chest radiograph **(E)** shows a severe scoliosis.

Such distorted architecture of the lung is a common finding in severe scoliosis.

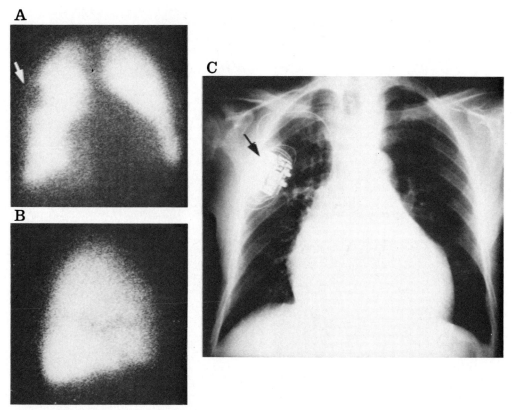

Case 4–8.—Pacemaker Artifact on a Perfusion Lung Scan

Perfusion lung scan obtained using technetium Tc-99m macroaggregated albumin on a 75-year-old man. Anterior image **(A)** shows a peripheral perfusion defect in the right upper lung *(arrow)*. The defect is not clearly seen on a right lateral view **(B).** The patient had a pacemaker implanted in his right anterior chest wall **(C)** that caused attenuation artifact on the perfusion image, a common artifact that appears on a perfusion lung scan.

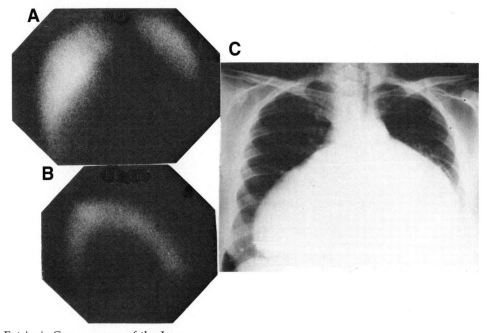

Case 4–9.—Extrinsic Compression of the Lung

Perfusion lung scan, anterior **(A)** and left lateral **(B)** views obtained with technetium Tc-99m macroaggregated albumin on a 34-year-old woman with long history of rheumatic heart disease, shows large perfusion defect in the right lower lung and only a rim of left upper lobe perfusion. A chest radiograph **(C)** taken on the day of the lung scan shows a massive cardiomegaly. Cardiomegaly and pleural effusion are the two most common causes of extrinsic compression of the lung resulting in perfusion defect on radionuclide lung images.

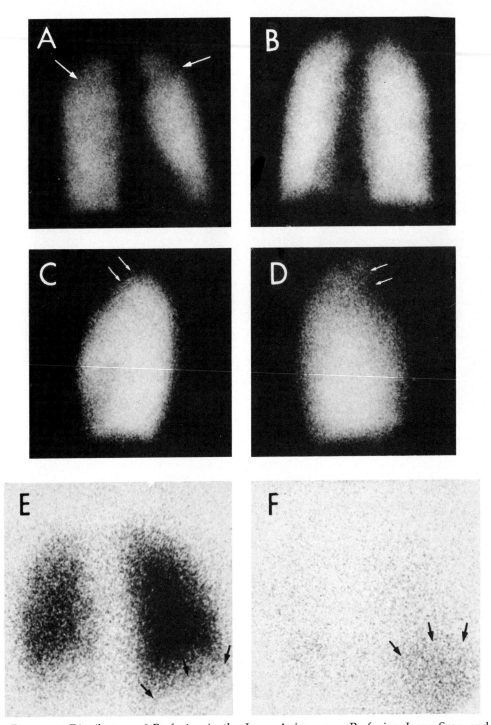

Case 4–10.—Decreased Distribution of Perfusion in the Lung Apices on a Perfusion Lung Scan and Retention of Xenon Xe 133 in the Liver on a Ventilation Lung Scan

Perfusion lung scan, anterior **(A)**, posterior **(B)**, and left **(C)** and right **(D)** lateral views obtained using technetium Tc-99m macroaggregated albumin show decreased perfusion distribution in the apices **(A,** *arrows*). This is a common finding on an anterior view, normal perfusion image. The finding is caused by smaller volume of the apices and apices far posteriorly located (distance from the gamma camera crystal) **(C** and **D,** *arrows*), and by attenuation by the clavicles and ribs.

The ventilation scan, an early equilibrium image **(E)** and two-minute washout image **(F),** show retention of the xenon Xe 133 in the liver **(F,** *arrows*).

Such xenon Xe 133 retention in the liver is a frequent finding on washout ventilation scans and should not lead to a false interpretation of an obstructive right lower lung disease. (Carey J.E., Purdy J.M., Moses D.C.: Localization of ^{133}Xe in liver during ventilation studies. *J. Nucl. Med.* 15:1179, 1974.)

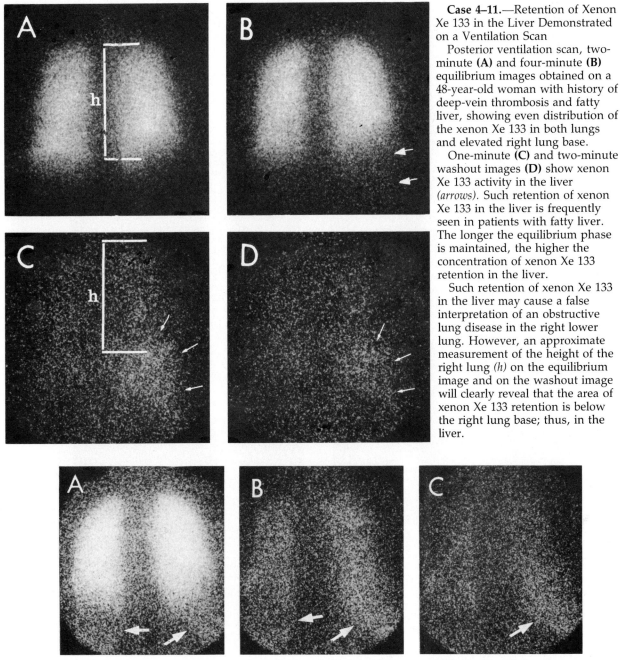

Case 4–11.—Retention of Xenon Xe 133 in the Liver Demonstrated on a Ventilation Scan

Posterior ventilation scan, two-minute **(A)** and four-minute **(B)** equilibrium images obtained on a 48-year-old woman with history of deep-vein thrombosis and fatty liver, showing even distribution of the xenon Xe 133 in both lungs and elevated right lung base.

One-minute **(C)** and two-minute washout images **(D)** show xenon Xe 133 activity in the liver *(arrows)*. Such retention of xenon Xe 133 in the liver is frequently seen in patients with fatty liver. The longer the equilibrium phase is maintained, the higher the concentration of xenon Xe 133 retention in the liver.

Such retention of xenon Xe 133 in the liver may cause a false interpretation of an obstructive lung disease in the right lower lung. However, an approximate measurement of the height of the right lung *(h)* on the equilibrium image and on the washout image will clearly reveal that the area of xenon Xe 133 retention is below the right lung base; thus, in the liver.

Case 4–12.—Xenon Xe 133 Localization in the Spleen and the Liver Demonstrated on a Ventilation Scan

Ventilation study performed using xenon Xe 133 on a 57-year-old man with sudden onset of shortness of breath. Posterior equilibrium image **(A)**, and 60-second **(B)** and 90-second **(C)** washout images show xenon Xe 133 activity in the liver and the spleen *(arrows)*.

The activity in the spleen was greatest on the equilibrium image and least on the 90-second washout image, while the activity in the liver remained relatively constant. A liver and spleen scan on this patient was normal.

The xenon Xe 133 retention in the liver is frequently seen, particularly in patients with fatty liver (Bianco J.A., Shafer R.B.: Implications of liver activity associated with ^{133}Xe ventilation lung scans. *Clin. Nucl. Med.* 3:176, 1976).

However, localization of xenon Xe 133 in the spleen has never been documented. The mechanism of the finding is not clear; however, faster clearance of the activity from the spleen than from the liver indicates that xenon Xe 133 localization in the spleen is not through exactly the same mechanism of the liver uptake.

This patient was receiving chemotherapy for his non-Hodgkin's lymphoma, and the change in the spleen caused by the chemotherapy may have contributed to the significant amount of xenon Xe 133 localization in the spleen.

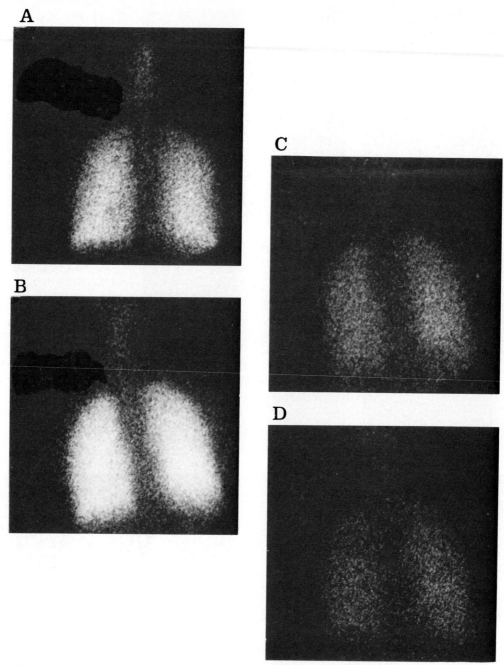

Case 4–13.—Delayed Xenon Xe 133 Washout in a Patient With Normal Lung Function

Ventilation study was performed using xenon Xe 133 on a 19-year-old girl with shortness of breath.

Single-breath image **(A)** and four-minute equilibrium image showed normal ventilation distribution. One-minute **(C)** and two-minute **(D)** washout images, however, showed abnormal retention of the xenon Xe 133 diffusely in both lungs. Other pulmonary function tests were all normal in this patient.

Such diffuse retention of xenon Xe 133 can occur in a patient without airway disease when the patient takes voluntary hypoventilation, often owing to the high oxygen content in the inhaling gas (xenon Xe 133 mixed in 95% oxygen) or to prolonged exposure—collection of certain counts on washout images instead of exposure for a given time, the same as that required for the equilibrium images.

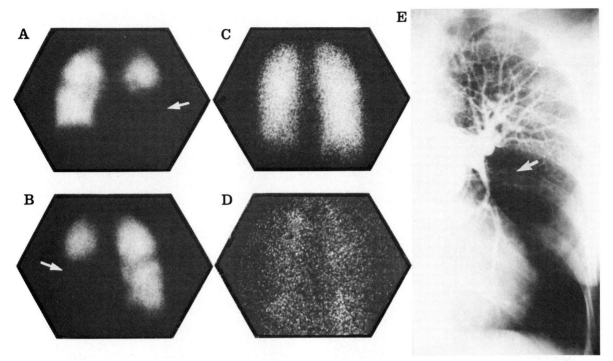

Case 4–14.—A Hypoplastic Pulmonary Artery Causing a Large Perfusion Defect Without Ventilation Defect

Perfusion lung scan, anterior **(A)** and posterior **(B)** views, obtained on a 9-year-old girl shows a large perfusion defect involving the lower two-thirds of the left lung.

Ventilation scan, posterior equilibrium **(C)** and washout **(D)** images, show no significant ventilation abnormality.

A left pulmonary angiogram **(E)** shows hypoplastic left pulmonary artery *(arrow)*.

This is a rare anomaly that is very likely to cause a false positive diagnosis of pulmonary embolism and can be diagnosed only by angiography.

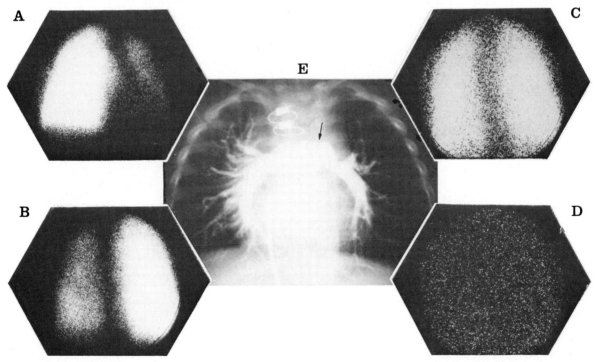

Case 4–15.—Aberrant Pulmonary Artery Causing Diffusely Decreased Perfusion on a Ventilation-Perfusion Lung Scan

Perfusion lung scan, anterior **(A)** and posterior **(B)** views obtained using technetium Tc-99m microspheres on a 14-month-old boy, shows diffusely decreased perfusion in the entire left lung.

A ventilation scan, posterior equilibrium **(C)** and washout **(D)** images, shows no ventilation abnormality.

The scan findings may suggest a left hilar mass lesion or left pulmonary artery thromboembolic process.

The patient had aberrant left pulmonary artery causing tracheal compression and diminished left pulmonary perfusion. Corrective surgery was performed; however, there was a severe stricture of the left pulmonary artery (**E,** *arrow*), causing the diffusely decreased distribution of perfusion.

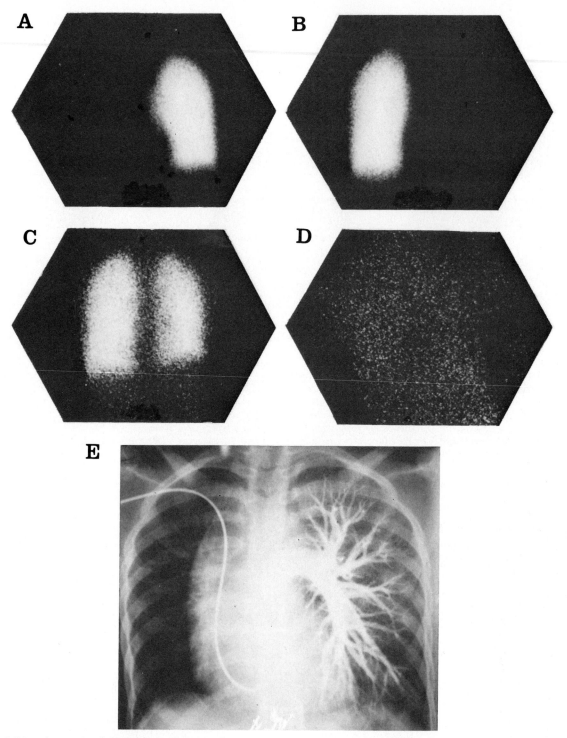

Case 4–16.—Agenesis of the Right Pulmonary Artery Causing Ventilation-Perfusion Mismatch Perfusion Defect of the Entire Lung

Anterior **(A)** and posterior **(B)** view perfusion lung scan obtained using technetium Tc-99m microspheres shows a total absence of perfusion in the right lung. Ventilation scan, posterior equilibrium **(C)** and washout images **(D)**, shows essentially normal ventilation. A main pulmonary artery angiogram **(E)** reveals agenesis of the right pulmonary artery.

This rare anomaly can be suspected from a chest radiograph with hyperlucency of a lung and shift of the mediastinum. The condition, however, may cause a false diagnosis of an obstruction of the pulmonary artery by a mediastinal or hilar mass lesion or an intrinsic obstruction by thromboembolic process. (Isawa T., Taplin G.V.: Unilateral pulmonary artery agenesis, and hypoplasia. *Radiology*, 99:605, 1971.)

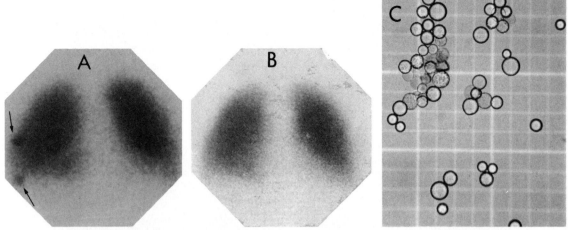

Case 4–17.—"Hot Spot" on a Perfusion Lung Scan; An Artifact Due to Poor-quality Radiopharmaceutical

Anterior perfusion lung scan **(A)** obtained using technetium Tc-99m microspheres shows two "hot spots," suspected to be due to poor preparation of the radiopharmaceutical. The remaining labeled particles, examined under a microscope **(C),** showed clumps of microspheres. A repeated anterior perfusion lung scan obtained the next day shows **(B)** normal perfusion distribution.

(Comments: When the labeling procedure of the technetium Tc-99m microspheres required boiling of the microsphere preparation, overheating occasionally occurred when the vial was left in a boiling water bath for longer than recommended. Such overheating caused clumping of the particle.)

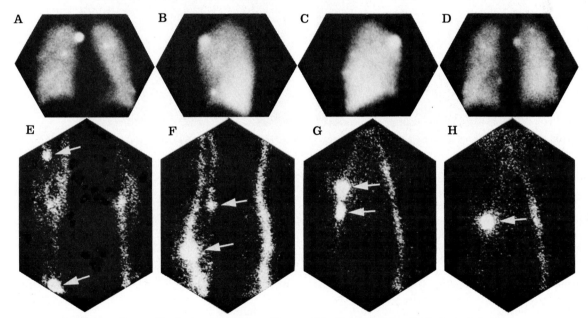

Case 4–18.—"Hot Spots" on a Perfusion Lung Scan Due to "Radioactive Clots"; Technical Artifact

Perfusion lung scan, anterior **(A),** left lateral **(B),** right lateral **(C),** and posterior views **(D),** obtained using technetium Tc-99m macroaggregated albumin on a 27-year-old woman with swollen right lower leg and chest pain shows multiple "hot spots" in both lungs. A lower extremity radionuclide venography was performed immediately before the lung scan and showed hot spots that were moving upward from the right lower leg (**E** to **H,** *arrows*). Because of the edema, intravenous injection was delayed, and, during the injection process, which took repeated attempts, aggregates of the blood and the technetium Tc-99m macroaggregated albumin apparently had formed in the vein and possibly in the syringe.

Such hot spots on a perfusion scan that were not caused by faulty injections have been reported in patients with thrombophlebitis (Lutzker L.G., Perez L.A.: Radioactive embolization from upper-extremity thrombophlebitis. *J. Nucl. Med.* 16:241, 1975), or with congestive heart failure (Goldberg E., Lieberman C.: "Hot spots" in lung scan. *J. Nucl. Med.* 18:499, 1977.)

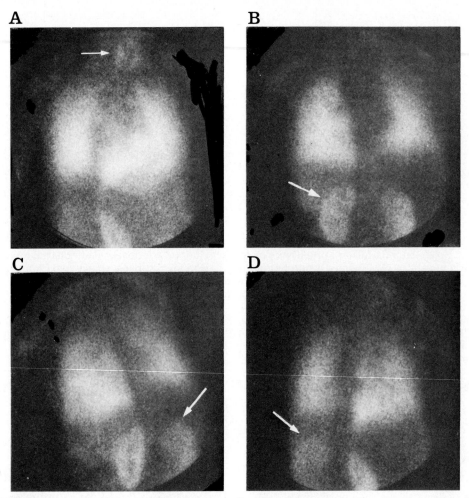

Case 4–19.—Visualization of Kidneys and Thyroid on a Perfusion Lung Scan; Poor Quality of Technetium Tc-99m Macroaggregated Albumin

Emergency perfusion lung scan obtained with technetium Tc-99m macroaggregated albumin, anterior **(A)**, posterior **(B)**, left posterior oblique **(C)**, and right posterior oblique **(D)** views, shows image of the kidneys and relatively high background activity. Such visualization of the kidneys on a perfusion lung scan commonly indicates the presence of right-to-left shunt.

Another frequent cause of the renal uptake has been a property of a commercial product, Tc-99m MAA (by Squibb & Sons Co.), that used to demonstrate image of the kidneys on perfusion lung scan. The mechanism of such localization in the kidney has never been clarified; however, 1.5%–22% of the injected dose could be found in the circulation immediately after the injection of technetium Tc-99m MAA (Blaufox M.D., Freeman L.M. (eds.): *Physicians Desk Reference For Radiology and Nuclear Medicine*. Oradell, New Jersey, Medical Economics Co., 1976–7, p. 142).

This activity, presumably unbound to macroaggregated albumin, could easily be localized in the kidney, or a large part of it should be excreted through the kidney. The product did not demonstrate visible thyroid uptake; therefore, the circulating activity probably did not represent free sodium pertechnetate Tc-99m.

In the case shown here, however, the anterior image **(A)** shows thyroid uptake *(arrow)* and the blood pool activity. Thus, the poor quality of the perfusion image was due to poor labeling of the technetium Tc-99m macroaggregated albumin.

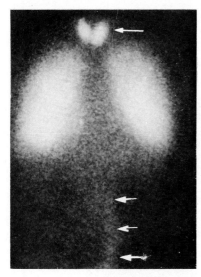

Case 4–20.—Inadequate Labeling of Technetium Tc-99m Macroaggregated Albumin: Free Pertechnetate Activity in the Lung Scanning Agent

Anterior view perfusion lung scan shows intense uptake by the thyroid gland *(long arrow)*. There is linear activity running in the abdomen, which probably represents aorta *(small arrows)*.

Cardiac silhouette is not clear, indicating radionuclide in the blood pool. These extrapulmonary activities indicate poorly labeled macroaggregated albumin with an unacceptably high amount of free Tc-99m pertechnetate.

Such poor-quality control results are often seen in cases of emergency lung scans performed during the weekend.

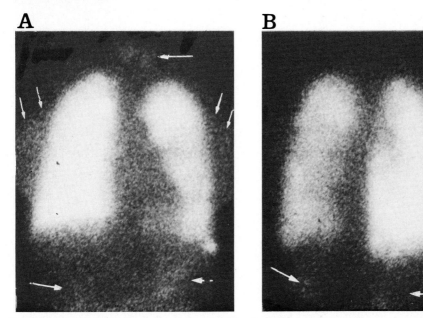

Case 4–21.—Poor-quality Perfusion Lung Scan Caused by Poorly Prepared Radiopharmaceutical

Emergency perfusion lung scan, anterior **(A)** and posterior **(B)** views, was obtained using technetium Tc-99m macroaggregated albumin on a 19-year-old woman with Sheehan's syndrome and shortness of breath.

The perfusion lung scan shows localization of radioactivity in the kidneys, breast, and thyroid gland *(arrows)*. Visualization of the kidney on a perfusion lung scan in general suggests right-to-left intracardiac shunt. However, when there is thyroid uptake, it means that the presence of free Tc-99m activity caused soft tissue and renal activity.

Such findings, along with a hot spot in the left anterior lung base, indicate poor radiopharmaceutical preparation and probable faulty injection—technical artifacts.

5

The Heart

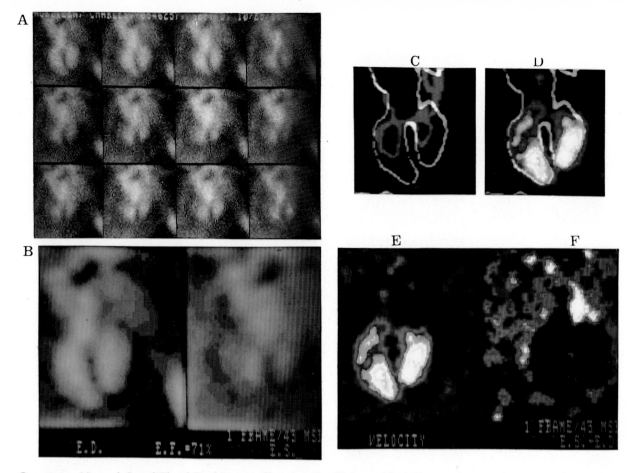

Case 5–1.—Normal Gated Blood Pool Images Showing the Right and Left Ventricular Functions in Various Means of Illustrations

A, gated blood pool images of the heart obtained at a 45° left anterior oblique view using technetium Tc-99m red blood cells labeled with in vivo labeling technique show both ventricles at different sequential, contraction-relaxation phases.

B, comparison of the ventricles at the end-diastolic phase *(E.D.)* and at the end-systolic phase *(E.S.)*. From the comparison, a physician can have a definite idea of the ventricular contraction status.

C, superimposition of the boundaries of the end-systole *(blue)* and end-diastole *(red)* ventricles. The *boundary lines* show status of regional wall motions.

D, functional image of the ventricles; kinetic image. The *bright areas* represent areas with active wall motion—vigorous wall contraction.

E, functional images of the ventricle. A velocity image, similar to the intensity image, shows velocity of the biventricular contraction. The brighter the area, the more efficient myocardial contraction it represents.

F, another functional image, dyskinesia image, a subtraction image that shows areas of ventricular dyskinesia as bright area. This patient obviously does not have dyskinesia.

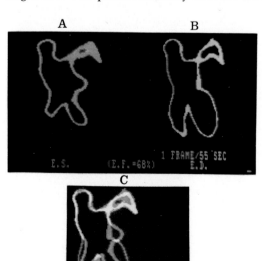

Case 5–2.—Boundary Line Image of the Gated Blood Pool Study

From the frames of the gated cardiac blood pool study, the frames with the smallest ventricular volume (**A,** *blue*) and the largest ventricular volume (**B,** *orange*) are selected and boundaries of the ventricles are displayed.

When the end-systolic and end-diastolic boundaries are superimposed (**C**), the image shows the normality of ventricular ejection fraction and regional wall motions.

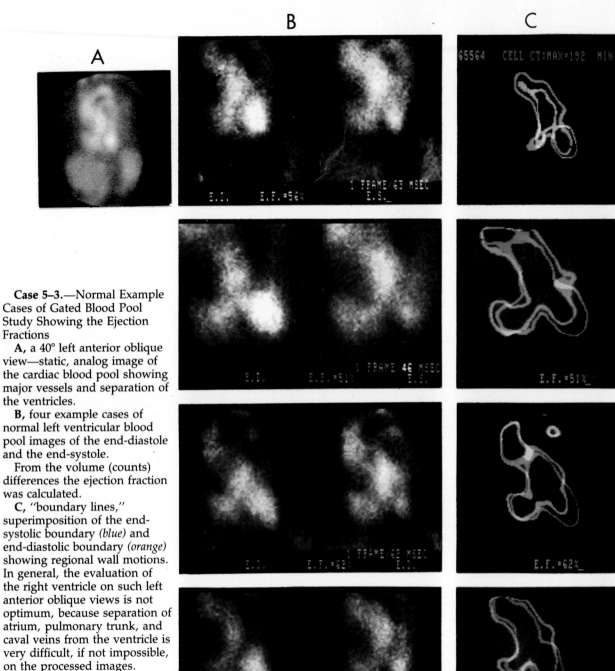

Case 5–3.—Normal Example Cases of Gated Blood Pool Study Showing the Ejection Fractions

A, a 40° left anterior oblique view—static, analog image of the cardiac blood pool showing major vessels and separation of the ventricles.

B, four example cases of normal left ventricular blood pool images of the end-diastole and the end-systole.

From the volume (counts) differences the ejection fraction was calculated.

C, "boundary lines," superimposition of the end-systolic boundary *(blue)* and end-diastolic boundary *(orange)* showing regional wall motions. In general, the evaluation of the right ventricle on such left anterior oblique views is not optimum, because separation of atrium, pulmonary trunk, and caval veins from the ventricle is very difficult, if not impossible, on the processed images.

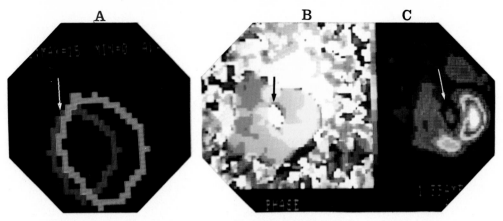

Case 5–4.—Septal Wall Dyskinesia or Akinesia on a Gated Blood Pool Study

Regional wall motion of the left ventricle, studied by means of gated blood pool images and displayed using boundary line image **(A),** shows dyskinesia of the septum *(arrow)*.

The septal dyskinesia is redemonstrated on phase image of the heart **(B)** and on a kinetic intensity image **(C).** The patient, however, had recently undergone coronary artery bypass surgery. The gated blood pool study invariably shows such septal dyskinesia or akinesia in a patient who has had cardiac surgery. The finding does not indicate a true septal abnormality, though the precise mechanism of such phenomena is not clear.

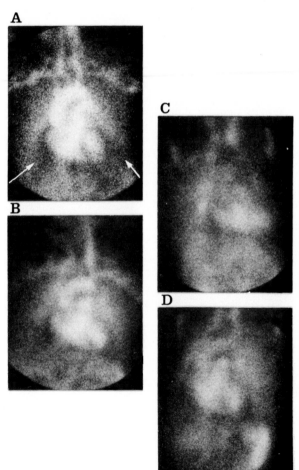

Case 5–5.—Effect of Positional Changes on a Cardiac Blood Pool Scan

Anterior image of the cardiac blood pool was obtained using technetium Tc-99m-labeled red blood cells on a 59-year-old man with congestive heart failure and suspected hemopericardium. An anterior image taken ten minutes after the injection **(A)** shows probable pericardial effusion *(arrows)*. A repeated anterior image was taken four hours later **(B),** showing no essential changes from the earlier image. Additional anterior view images were taken at a left decubitus position **(C)** and right decubitus position **(D)** to demonstrate shift of the pericardial fluid. The decubitus positions caused marked changes in the position and rotation of the heart. The anterior view at the left decubitus shows mainly the right heart; the left heart and the aortic arch are not well delineated. On the anterior view at the right decubitus, the main pulmonary trunk is best demonstrated. Separation of the right and left ventricles is best seen on the supine anterior images in this patient.

(Comment: the heart is an organ which changes its axis, rotation, and position more than other organs upon changes in patient's position. Therefore, proper positioning of the patient is the first important step to ensure effective and good-quality radionuclide cardiac studies.)

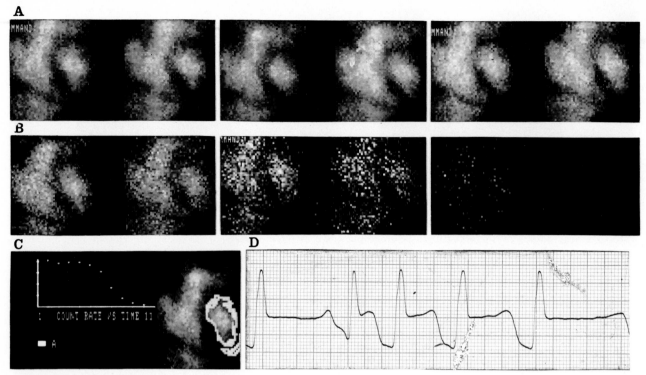

Case 5–6.—Severe Arrhythmia May Invalidate Gated Blood Pool Study

Multigated blood pool study obtained using technetium Tc-99m red blood cells labeled using the in vivo technique shows good-quality images of the ventricles in the earlier phase **(A).** However, the blood pool images fade gradually in the later phase **(B).**

The left ventricular volume curve shows no relaxation phase **(C).** ECG on the patient obtained during the study shows very irregular cardiac **(D)** rhythm.

In a patient with such markedly irregular cardiac rhythm, a conventional multigated blood pool study cannot effectively evaluate the cardiac function, even with an arrhythmia-filtering computer program, and can generate false values of the ejection fraction. True ejection fraction changes beat by beat when there is arrhythmia. First-pass technique and list mode acquisition of cardiac cycles may effectively be used in such patients.

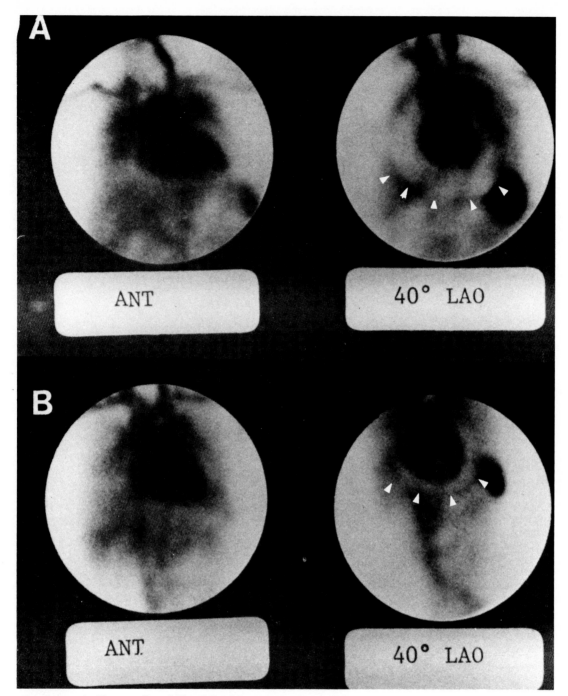

Case 5–7.—Breast Artifact on Gated Blood Pool Images

A, gated blood pool study on a 52-year-old woman admitted for congestive heart failure; 40° left anterior oblique view *(right)* shows evidence of a massive pericardial effusion *(arrows)*. The anterior view *(left)*, however, shows no evidence of effusion. The artifactitious "effusion" was caused by the large breast-attenuating background activities.

B, gated blood pool study on a 45-year-old woman with left bundle-branch block and first-degree atrioventricular block; 40° left anterior oblique view with 15° caudad tilt *(right)* shows "halo" around the heart, indicating possible pericardial effusion *(arrows)*. The anterior view *(left)*, however, shows no evidence of effusion, another example case of the breast tissue attenuation causing artifactitious pericardial effusion.

(Courtesy of Meyer-Pavel C., Clark J.K., Pavel D.G. [University of Illinois Medical Center, Chicago]: Incidence and consequences of breast artifacts in radionuclide cardiac studies. *Clin. Nucl. Med.* 7:53, 1982. Used by permission.)

A

B

C

Case 5–8.—Free Sodium
Pertechnetate Tc-99m Activity on
Blood Pool Images With in vivo-
Labeled Tc-99m Red Blood Cells;
Radiopharmaceutical Artifact

Anterior **(left row)** and posterior
(right row) views of blood pool
images over the chest and
abdomen were obtained 5 minutes
(A), 20 minutes **(B),** and 60
minutes **(C)** after the in vivo
labeling procedure (Pavel D.G.,
Zimmer A.M., Patterson V.N.: In
vivo labeling of red blood cells
with ^{99m}Tc: A new approach to
blood pool visualization. *N. Nucl.
Med.* 18:305, 1977) on a 54-year-old
woman with a suspected
hemangioma of the liver. In
addition to normal blood pool in
the heart, spleen, and great
vessels, the anterior images show
collection of radioactivity in the
stomach *(thin arrows)* and right
renal pelvis **(A,** *arrowhead).*

The radionuclide in the stomach
changes its location, indicating a
passage into the duodenum **(B**
and **C,** *arrows).* Such findings are
commonly seen in patients with in
vivo-labeled ^{99m}Tc-99m RBCs and
indicate that the technique has
shortcomings, with considerable
amount of free sodium
pertechnetate Tc-99m remaining
unbound. In our experience, on
the average 15% of the injected
sodium pertechnetate Tc-99m
remains unbound to the RBCs.
Arrowheads on the posterior views
(B and **C)** indicate small
hemangioma (2.5 cm) in the
posterior liver.

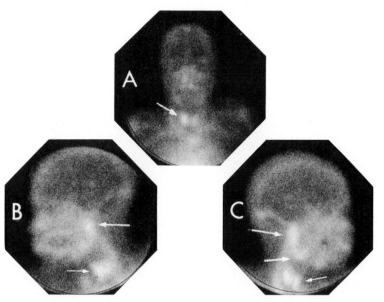

Case 5–9.—Free Pertechnetate Activity on Blood Pool Images With Technetium Tc-99m-labeled Red Blood Cells; Radiopharmaceutical Artifact

Anterior **(A)**, left **(B)** and right **(C)** lateral views of the head and neck obtained on a 35-year-old woman with congestive heart failure after a gated blood pool study. The images show the radionuclide distribution to be mainly in the blood pool. However, there is prominent uptake by the thyroid *(thin arrow)* and salivary glands *(thick arrows)*, indicating that significant amount of free sodium pertechnetate Tc-99m remained in the circulation after the in vivo RBC-labeling process.

The in vivo labeling technique allows about 15% of the injected activity to remain unbound, as free sodium pertechnetate Tc-99m.

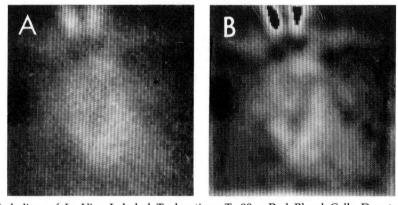

Case 5–10.—Poor Labeling of In Vivo-Labeled Technetium Tc-99m Red Blood Cells Due to Intravenous Heparin; Radiopharmaceutical Artifact

Digital images of an anterior cardiac blood pool, without **(A)** and with nine-point smoothing **(B),** obtained using the in vivo-labeled technetium Tc-99m RBCs, show extremely poor resolution of the cardiac chambers, high background activity, and highest activity in the thyroid gland. The findings indicate very poor labeling of the RBCs and high free sodium pertechnetate Tc-99m activity.

The patient, a 54-year-old man with recent myocardial infarction and pulmonary embolism, had received a high dose of intravenous heparin. It has been a frequent experience that intravenous heparin at high doses interferes with the efficacy of the in vivo-labeling procedure of the technetium Tc-99m RBCs. Such interference of labeling by the heparin, however, is not a universal experience, and the mechanism of the effect of the heparin has not been documented, though a certain antihypertensive drug has been reported to influence the labeling efficiency of technetium Tc-99m red blood cells. (Lee H.B., Wexler J.P., Scharf S.C., et al.: Pharmacologic alterations in Tc-99m binding by red blood cells: Concise communication. *J. Nucl. Med.* 24:397, 1983.)

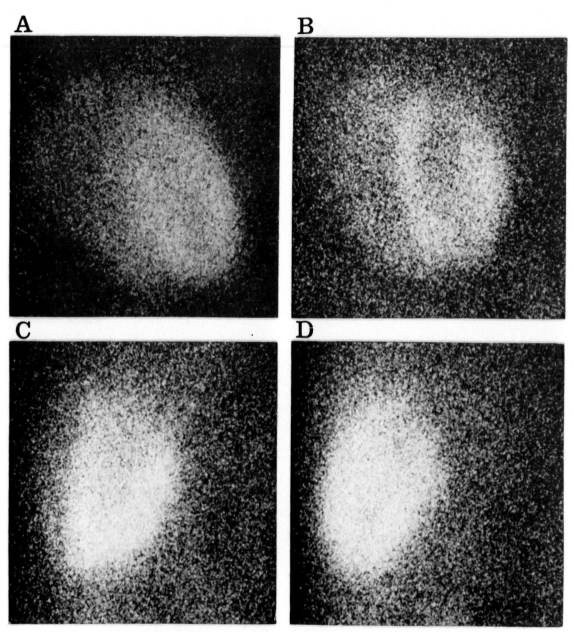

Case 5–11.—Example of Vertical Heart on an Exercise Thallous Chloride Tl 201 Scan

Exercise thallium 201 scan obtained on a 39-year-old woman with chest pain, anterior **(A),** 35° **(B)** and 70° **(C)** left anterior oblique, and left lateral **(D)** views, shows almost vertical axis of the left ventricle with normal distribution of the thallium 201, a normal variant frequently seen in athletic individuals and thin patients.

The patient had normal exercise ECG and enzyme studies.

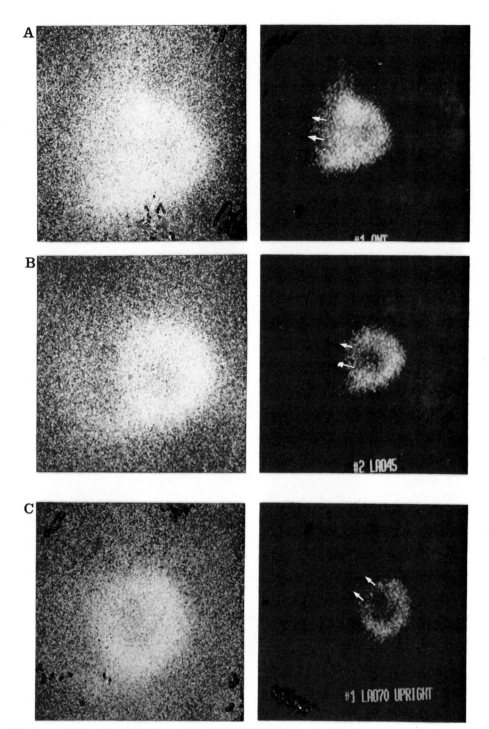

Case 5–12.—Horizontal Heart on a Thallous Chloride Tl 201 Scan

Thallium 201 myocardial images, anterior **(A)** and 45° left anterior oblique **(B)** views, obtained immediately after a treadmill exercise. Analog images **(left column)** and digital images **(right column)** show the heart to be in a horizontal position with the outflow tract directed toward the right side instead of upward *(arrows)*. Left anterior oblique view, 70°, taken at upright position **(C)** shows a significant change in the axis of the heart, the outflow tract pointing almost upward *(arrows)*.

Horizontal heart is more frequently noted in elderly or overweight individuals and may cause false interpretation of the outflow tract as an ischemic area.

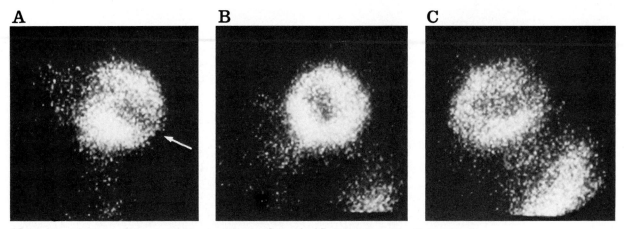

Case 5–13.—A Normal "Apical Thinning" on an Exercise Thallous Chloride Tl 201 Study

Digital images of an exercise thallium 201 scan. Anterior **(A),** 45° left anterior oblique **(B),** and left lateral **(C)** views show decreased activity in the apex. This appearance of apical defect is seen on the anterior view *(arrow),* only barely on the lateral view, and not on the oblique view.

Such apical thinning has been reported in over 50% of normal hearts, though the exact cause of the "normal apical defect" has not been documented (Cook D.J., Bailey I., Strauss H.W., et al.: Thallium-201 for myocardial imaging: Appearance of the normal heart. *J. Nucl. Med.* 17:583, 1976).

Case 5–14.—"Full Stomach" on "Heavy Meal" Sign on a Thallous Chloride Tl 201 Scan

Exercise thallium-201 scan, analog *(left)* and digital *(right)* images of anterior **(A)** and left lateral view **(B)** obtained on a 43-year-old, 210-lb woman shows a large photon-deficient area below the left ventricle *(arrows),* representing a full stomach.

The heart is in the horizontal position on the anterior view. The border of the inferior wall appears to be irregular on the lateral view.

These findings are due to a full stomach, which pushes up the apex causing the horizontal heart and attenuation on the inferior wall.

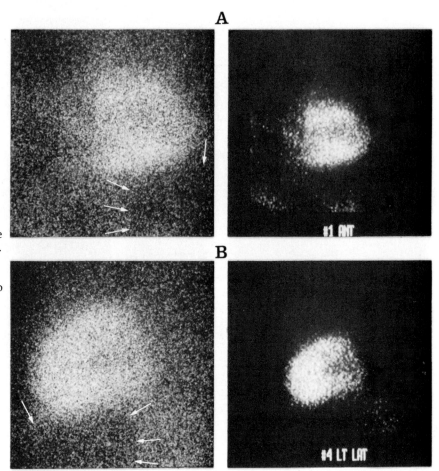

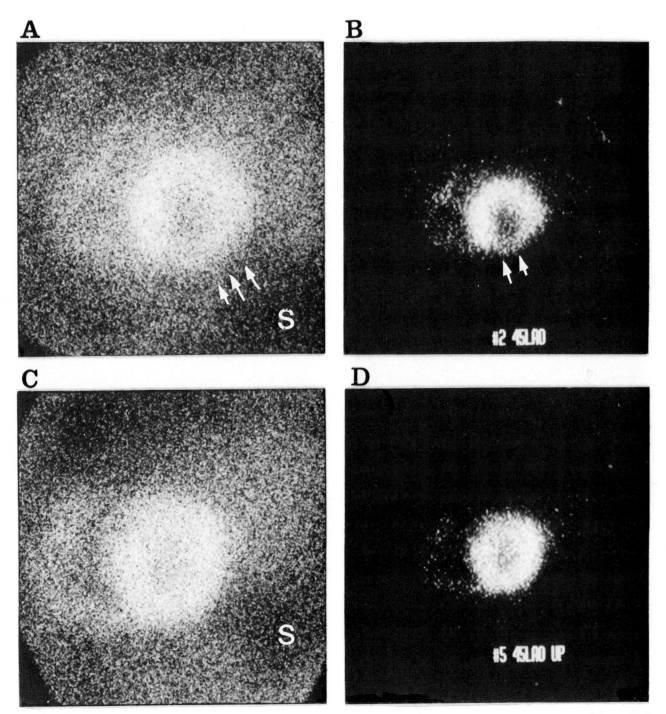

Case 5–15.—Artifactitious Defect-Attenuation Artifact on an Exercise Thallous Chloride Tl 201 Scan Caused by a "Full Stomach"

Exercise thallium-201 scan obtained on a 65-year-old woman. 45° left anterior oblique view of analog **(A)** and digital **(B)** images show abnormally decreased perfusion in the inferoapical wall *(arrows)*. In addition, a large photon-deficient area is noted below the left ventricle *(S)*, representing a full stomach.

Repeated images obtained at upright position **(C** and **D)** show normal thallium-201 distribution in the inferoapical wall.

The initial artifactitious defect is caused by attenuation by the diaphragm, more frequently seen in patients with a full stomach.

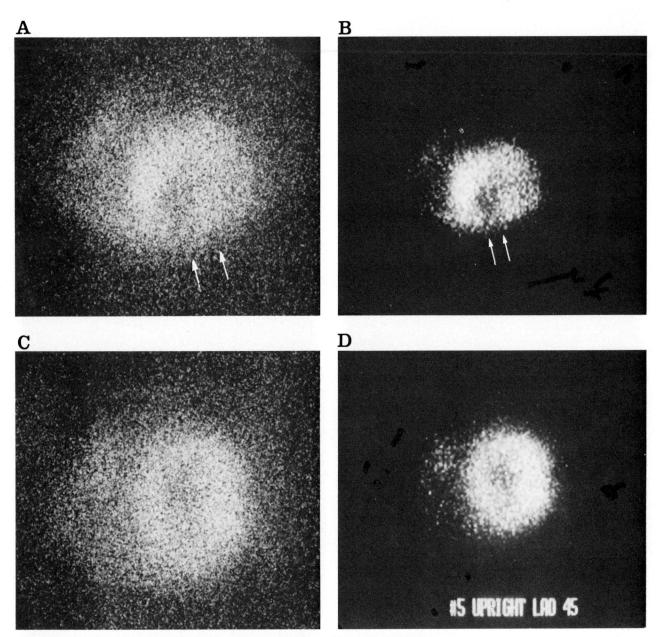

A **B**

C **D**

#5 UPRIGHT LAO 45

Case 5–16.—Attenuation Artifact on an Exercise Thallous Chloride Tl 201 Scan

Analog **(A)** and digital **(B)** images of an exercise thallium 201 scan. 45° left anterior oblique view at supine position obtained on a 54-year-old man without risk factors shows a focal area of decreased thallium-201 distribution *(arrows)* in the inferoapical wall.

Immediately the view was repeated at upright position **(C and D),** and the inferoapical wall showed a normal distribution of thallium-201.

Such artifactitious defect in the inferoapical wall is seen frequently on a thallium-201 image taken at supine position. Attenuation artifact on a thallium-201 scan commonly is caused by the breast or diaphragm. (Botvinick E.H., Dunn R.F., Hattner R.S., et al.: A consideration of factors affecting the diagnostic accuracy of thallium-201 myocardial perfusion scintigraphy in detecting coronary artery disease. *Semin. Nucl. Med.* 10:157, 1980.) When such a defect is noted on "one view only," the view should be repeated at supine position. True lesion appears on more than one view in most cases.

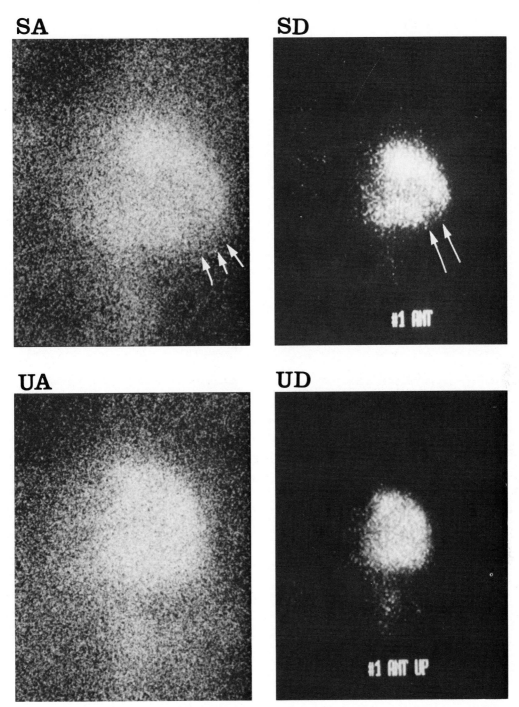

SA

SD

#1 ANT

UA

UD

#1 ANT UP

Case 5–17.—Attenuation Artifact on a Thallous Chloride Tl-201 Myocardial Scan and Positional Changes

Anterior view analog **(SA)** and digital **(SD)** images of an exercise thallium-201 myocardial perfusion scan obtained at supine position on a 60-year-old woman with a history of myocardial infarction shows a focal defect in the apical-inferior wall *(arrows).* An immediately obtained repeated view at upright position, analog **(UA)** and digital **(UD)** images, shows essentially normal apical and inferior wall.

The defect seen on the initial supine scan was an attenuation artifact caused by the stomach and diaphragm. An immediate, repeated scan at upright position is the most useful technique to differentiate a true perfusion defect from an attenuation artifact.

The stomach *(s)* is noted as a photon-deficient area on the initial anterior image and is shifted away in the repeated upright image.

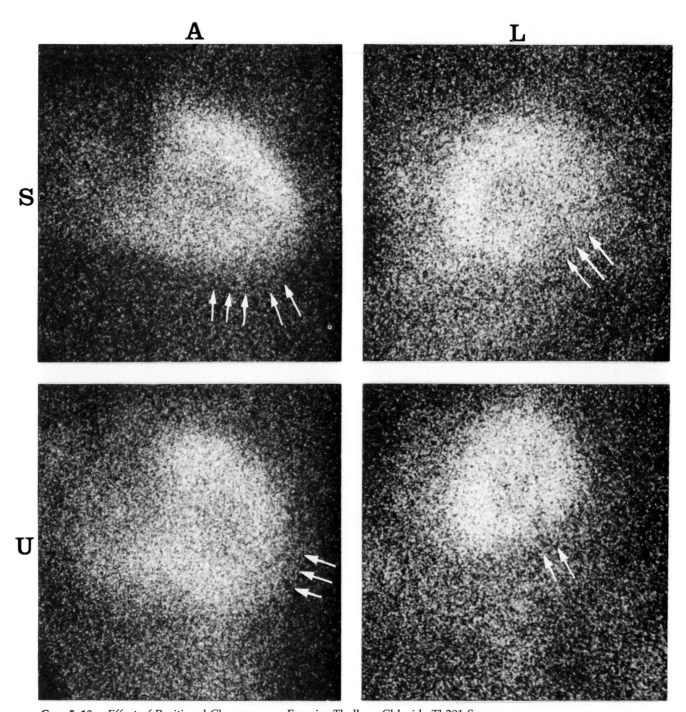

A

L

S

U

Case 5–18.—Effect of Positional Change on an Exercise Thallous Chloride Tl 201 Scan

Exercise thallium 201 scans, anterior **(A)** and 70° left anterior oblique views **(L),** show a diffusely decreased activity in the inferior wall **(A,** *arrows*) and posterolateral wall **(L,** *arrows*).

Immediately the same views were repeated at upright position **(U).** The areas of decreased activity changed their size and locations on the upright images *(arrows).* When there is artifactitious defect on an exercise thallium 201 scan owing to tissue attenuation by stomach, diaphragm, or breast, etc., the defect changes its size and/or location when a repeated image is taken at upright position—a very effective technique to reduce the incidence of false positive thallium 201 scan results.

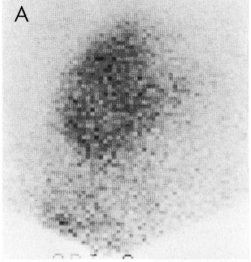

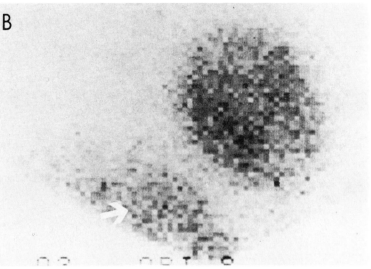

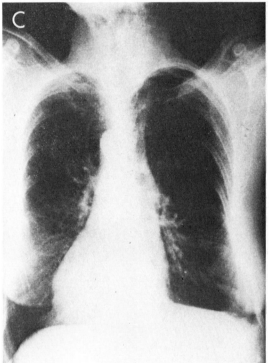

Case 5–19.—Situs Inversus; Imaging of the Heart With Thallous Chloride Tl 201 in Patient With Situs Inversus

A: Anterior view thallium 201 image of the heart; dextrocardia. The image mimics a left lateral view of a normally positioned heart.

B: Left anterior oblique view, 45°, of the dextrocardia. The activity in the liver is seen in the left abdomen *(white arrow).*

C: Chest radiograph of the patient with situs inversus.

(Courtesy of Kasner J.R., Kamrani F. [Good Samaritan Medical Center, Milwaukee, Wisconsin]: Thallium imaging in a patient with situs inversus. *Clin. Nucl. Med.* 8:224, 1983.)

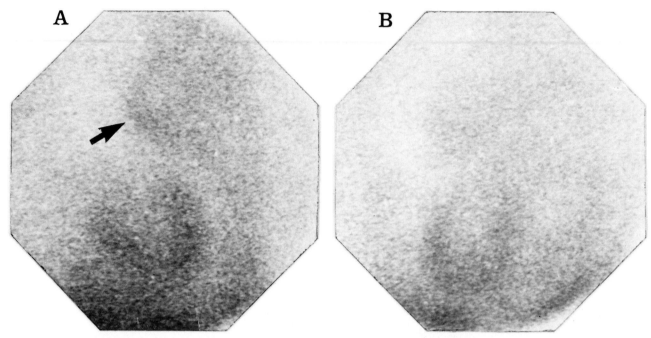

Case 5–20.—Demonstration of a Lung Carcinoma on a Thallous Chloride Tl 201 Myocardial Scan

Resting myocardial scan with thallium 201, anterior **(A)** and 70° left anterior oblique **(B)** views, obtained on a 50-year-old man with suspected myocardial infarction shows a normal left ventricular uptake.

In addition, another round rim activity in the shape of a heart is noted above the ventricle *(arrow)*. The extracardiac uptake represented an anaplastic carcinoma in the patient's left upper lung.

When a thallium 201 myocardial scan is performed in a patient with a tumor nearby the heart attention is needed to obtain proper image of the heart. There might be a misleading uptake by a tumor that may be superimposed on or adjacent to the heart.

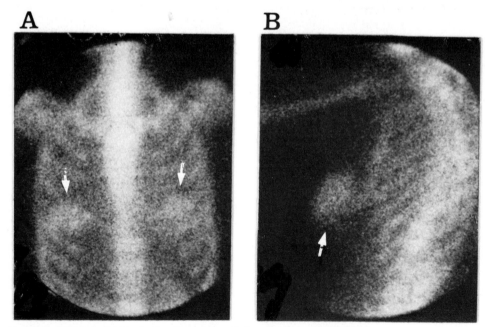

Case 5–21.—Small But Metabolically Active Breast Localizing the Bone-imaging Agent

Anterior view thoracic bone scan obtained using technetium Tc 99m pyrophosphate **(A)** shows small areas of uptake in the bilateral chest wall *(arrows)*. A left lateral view **(B)** shows the uptake to be in the breast *(arrows)*. Because of the localization of the bone-imaging agent by the breast tissue, it frequently interferes with effective evaluation of a myocardial scan with technetium Tc 99m pyrophosphate.

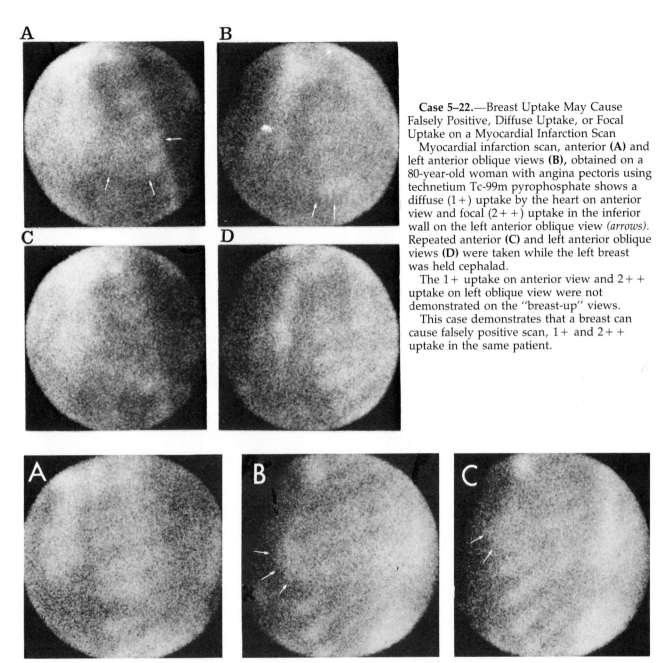

Case 5–22.—Breast Uptake May Cause Falsely Positive, Diffuse Uptake, or Focal Uptake on a Myocardial Infarction Scan

Myocardial infarction scan, anterior **(A)** and left anterior oblique views **(B)**, obtained on a 80-year-old woman with angina pectoris using technetium Tc-99m pyrophosphate shows a diffuse (1+) uptake by the heart on anterior view and focal (2++) uptake in the inferior wall on the left anterior oblique view *(arrows)*. Repeated anterior **(C)** and left anterior oblique views **(D)** were taken while the left breast was held cephalad.

The 1+ uptake on anterior view and 2++ uptake on left oblique view were not demonstrated on the "breast-up" views.

This case demonstrates that a breast can cause falsely positive scan, 1+ and 2++ uptake in the same patient.

Case 5–23.—Small Breast Uptake That May be Indistinguishable From Focal, Myocardial Uptake

Myocardial infarction scan, anterior **(A)** and left lateral views **(B)**, obtained on a 72-year-old woman with suspected myocardial infarction using technetium Tc-99m pyrophosphate shows abnormally increased uptake in the apical region **(B**, *arrows)*. A repeated lateral view was taken while her small breast was retracted upward.

The repeated scan shows the focal uptake to be less prominent and moved upward, demonstrating that a small breast uptake may mimic a focal myocardial uptake.

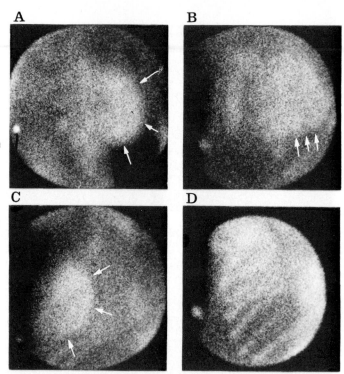

Case 5–24.—Uptake by the Breast May Cause Falsely Positive Findings of Massive Myocardial Infarction on a Myocardial Scan

Myocardial infarction scan was obtained on a 44-year-old woman with history of myocardial infarction and recent onset of chest pain, using technetium Tc-99m pyrophosphate. A left anterior oblique view **(B)** and left lateral view **(C)** show a large area of abnormal uptake that is attributable to a massive myocardial uptake infarction *(arrows).*

The anterior view **(A),** however, shows the intense uptake to be not in the region of the heart but in the large left breast *(arrows).* The left lateral view was repeated while the breast was held cephalad. The repeated lateral view **(D)** scan shows no abnormal uptake in the heart.

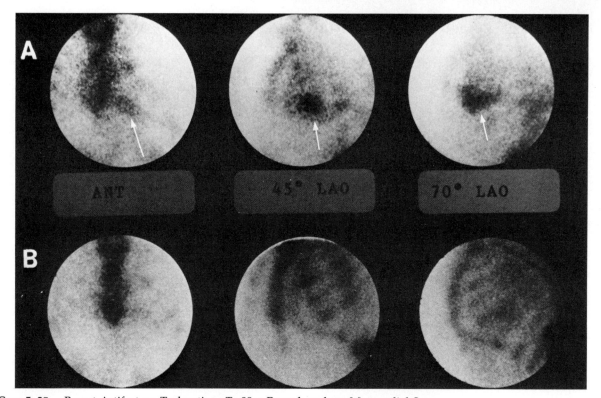

Case 5–25.—Breast Artifact on Technetium Tc-99m Pyrophosphate Myocardial Scan

Technetium Tc-99m pyrophosphate myocardial scans of 72-year-old woman with chest pain but without ECG changes. **A:** Scan at two hours postinjection shows marked discrete uptake in area of myocardium. **B:** At five hours postinjection, the discrete uptake disappeared. Absence of myocardial infarction was confirmed by serial ECG and CPK-MB enzyme studies.

(Courtesy of Meyer-Pavel C., Clark J.K., Pavel D.G. [University of Illinois Medical Center, Chicago]: Incidence and consequences of breast artifacts in radionuclide cardiac studies. *Clin. Nucl. Med.* 7:53, 1982.)

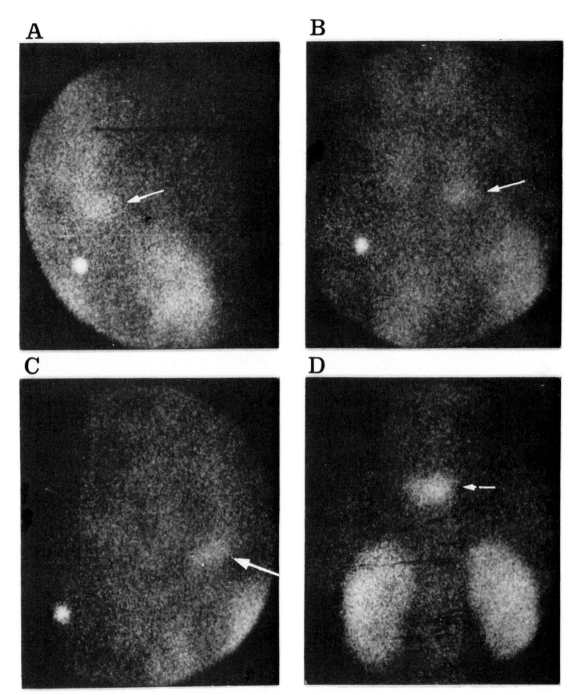

Case 5–26.—Abnormal Bone Lesion in a Thoracic Vertebra May Cause a Falsely Positive Myocardial Infarction Scan.

Myocardial infarction scan, anterior **(A),** 30° left anterior oblique **(B),** and 70° left anterior oblique **(C)** views, was obtained on a 63-year-old woman with recent ECG changes, using technetium Tc-99m pyrophosphate. The scans show focal abnormal uptake; however, the focus of the uptake cannot be precisely correlated with a myocardial region *(arrows)*; posterior view shows the abnormal uptake to be in a thoracic vertebra, T-10 **(D,** *arrow)*. An intense uptake by the kidneys is also noted.

When an area of abnormal uptake changes its location on different views, it most likely represents an artifactitious lesion on a myocardial scan.

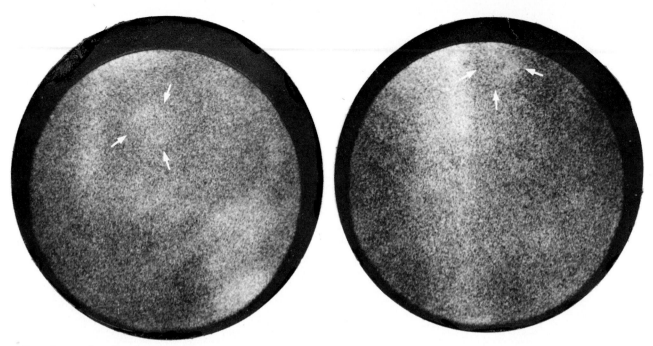

Case 5–27.—Localization of Technetium Tc-99m Pyrophosphate in the Subcutaneous Tissue Surrounding Implanted Pacemaker

Myocardial infarction scan obtained using a 15-mCi dose of technetium Tc-99m pyrophosphate on a 73-year-old woman showed a round area of abnormal uptake *(arrows)*. Precise localization of the uptake in relation to the heart could not be made on the 45° left anterior oblique view **(left)**. The anterior view **(right),** however, showed the area of abnormal uptake to be high in the anterior chest, higher than the level of the heart.

The patient had an implanted chest wall pacemaker corresponding to the area of abnormal uptake.

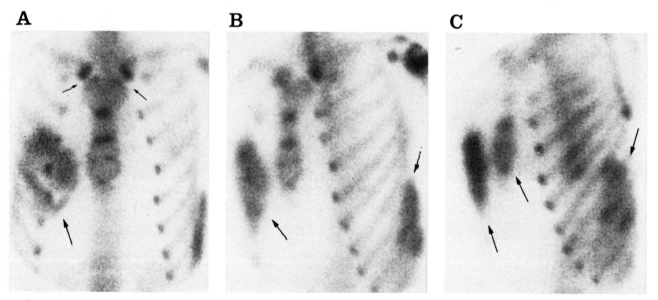

Case 5–28.—Images of the Chest Wall Injuries and Trauma of the Sternum on a Myocardial Infarction Scan

Myocardial infarction scan, anterior **(A),** 45° **(B)** and 70° **(C)** anterior oblique views, obtained using technetium Tc-99m pyrophosphate shows areas of abnormally increased uptake in the right anterior chest wall, distal sternum, sternoclavicular junction, and left lower lateral chest wall *(arrows)*. The appearance and location of the findings indicate burn injuries of chest wall from an electrical cardioversion and fracture of distal sternum from the cardiac resuscitation. Dislocation with increased uptake is obvious in the sternoclavicular junction **(A,** *arrows)*, also indicating trauma from the resuscitation procedure.

Locations of these areas of uptake are away from the heart; thus, they may not cause a false positive scan interpretation. When such soft tissue injury occurs in the chest wall in front of or near the heart, it may cause false interpretations. (Davison R., Spies S.M., Przybylek J, et al.: Technetium-99m-stannous pyrophosphate myocardial scintigraphy after cardiopulmonary resuscitation with cardioversion. *Circulation* 60:292, 1979.)

6

The Liver and Spleen

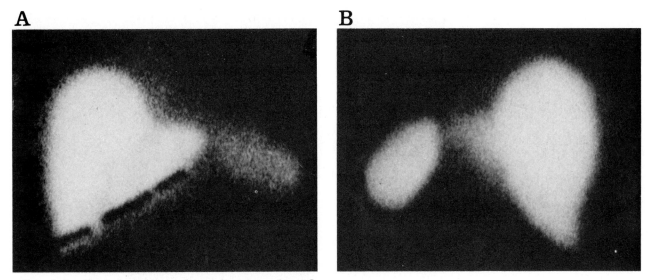

Case 6–1.—Typical *en chapeau des gendarme* on a Liver Scan

Liver and spleen scan, anterior **(A)** and posterior **(B)** views obtained using technetium Tc-99m sulfur colloid, shows a high dome of the liver with straight inferior border, forming the typical "policeman's hat" described by French authors (Caroli J., Bonneville B.: Diagnostic value of hepatic scintillography, *Arch. Mal Appar. Dig.* 51:55, 1962).

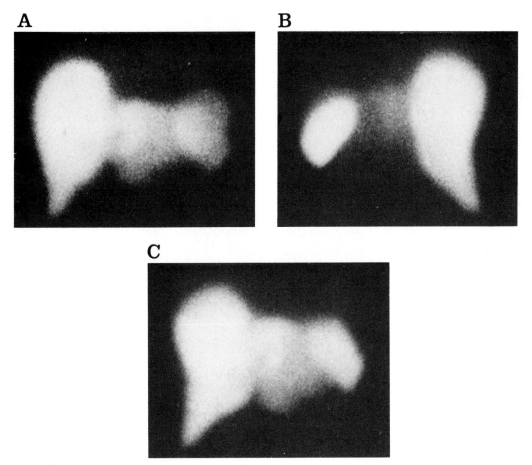

Case 6–2.—High Dome of the Liver

Anterior **(A)** and posterior **(B)** images of the liver and spleen at supine position obtained using technetium Tc-99m sulfur colloid show an unusually elevated dome of the liver.

Such findings have been described as results of a high diaphragm, seen in 14% of liver scans (McAfee J.G., Ause R.G., Wagner H.N.; Diagnostic value of scintillation scanning of the liver. *Arch. Intern. Med.* 116:95, 1965).

When a repeated anterior image was obtained at upright position **(C)**, the high dome became less obvious.

This patient had no pathological process in the right lung or in the diaphragm.

Case 6–3.—Normal Location of the Liver Shown on Anterior Liver Scan

Three examples of normal anterior liver images obtained using technetium Tc-99m sulfur colloid showing the right costal margin and the liver. Rarely, the inferior border of the liver lies above the right costal margin. When the anterior image is taken at upright position, the inferior border of a normal liver may extend 5–8 cm below the costal margin.

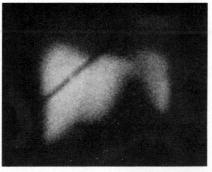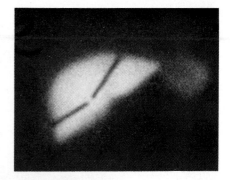

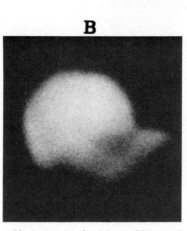

The criterion for a hepatomegaly must be based strictly on the vertical and transverse diameter of the liver, and the position of the patient at the time of imaging should be considered before one gives significance to a hepatomegaly or displacement of the liver.

A **B** **C**

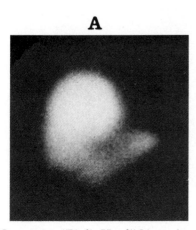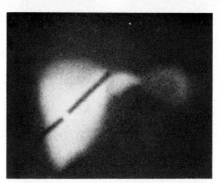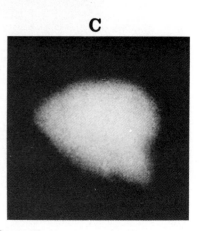

Case 6–4.—"Bird's Head" Liver; Another Variation in the Normal Liver Configuration

Anterior **(A),** right anterior oblique **(B),** and right lateral views **(C)** of a liver scan obtained using technetium Tc-99m sulfur colloid show very high dome of the right lobe and extremely small left lobe of the liver, forming a shape of a "bird's head" or a "baseball hat."

This variant may be regarded as an extreme form of "policeman's hat" shape of the liver (McAfee J.G., Ause R.G., Wagner H.N.: Diagnostic value of scintillation scanning of the liver. *Arch. Intern. Med.* 116:95, 1965).

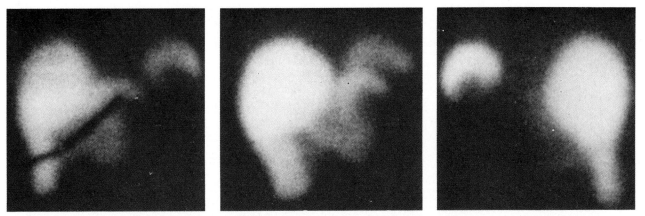

Case 6–5.—Liver and Spleen in an Appearance of a Turkey; Another Normal Variant on a Liver and Spleen Scan

Liver and spleen scan, supine anterior **(A)**, upright anterior **(B)**, and posterior **(C)** views, obtained using technetium Tc-99m sulfur colloid on a 72-year-old woman shows unusually deformed liver and spleen on the anterior views. The left lobe appears to be displaced toward the right, and the spleen is displaced upward. Such deformation of the liver and spleen is commonly caused by the stomach if there has been a long history of bulky food ingestion.

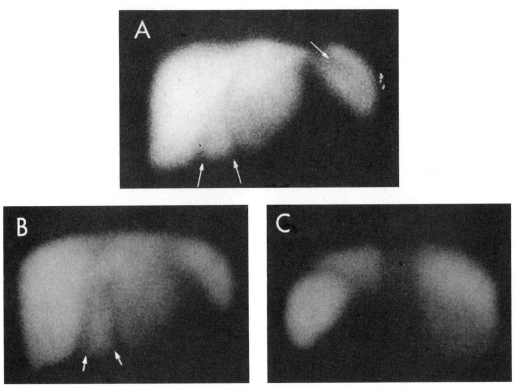

Case 6–6.—Caudate Lobe of the Liver on a Liver and Spleen Scan

Liver and spleen scan obtained on a 61-year-old man with colon carcinoma using technetium Tc-99m sulfur colloid shows a prominent caudate lobe of the liver. The initial anterior image taken at supine position **(A)** shows the caudate lobe *(arrows)* and prominent hilus of the spleen *(thin arrow)*.

A repeated anterior view at upright position delineated the caudate lobe more clearly (**B,** *arrows*). Owing to the change of position, the left lobe of the liver also became more prominent and thinner. The spleen is slightly rotated medially and inferiorly; thus, the hilus is no longer visible. **C,** posterior image of the liver and spleen at upright position.

(Comments: the caudate lobe of the liver receives arterial supply from both the right and left hepatic artery branches and venous drainage through both branches in 70% of cases. Thus, the lobe frequently is spared from extensive thromboembolic disease of the liver. Meindok H., Langer B.: Liver scan in Budd-Chiari syndrome. *J. Nucl. Med.* 17:365, 1976).

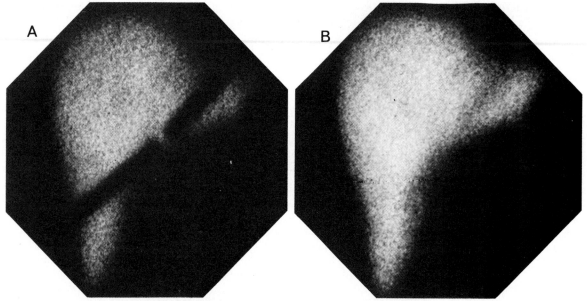

Case 6–7.—Riedel's Lobe of the Liver

Anterior liver images with **(A)** or without **(B)** costal lead marker were obtained using a 4-mCi dose of technetium Tc-99m sulfur colloid. The images show an elongated right lobe of the liver and almost absent, very small left lobe of the liver. The liver is otherwise essentially normal.

(Comment: the Riedel's lobe of the liver described in the early radiological imaging literature appeared as an abnormally enlarged right lobe of the liver or an accessory lobe of the liver attached to the inferior right lobe. [Lipchik E.O., Schwartz S.I.: Angiographic and scintillographic identification of Riedel's lobe of the liver. *Radiology* 88:48, 1967]. The figure shown here, however, represents a typical, normal Riedel's lobe of the liver.)

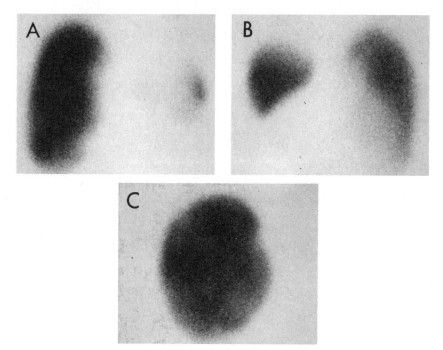

Case 6–8.—Another Form of the Riedel's Lobe of the Liver

Anterior **(A)**, posterior **(B)**, and right lateral **(C)** views of the liver and spleen scan obtained using technetium Tc-99m sulfur colloid on a 67-year-old man with suspected colon carcinoma show absent left lobe of the liver, with enlarged, thick right lobe of the liver. The finding is highly suggestive of metastatic disease that replaced the left lobe; however, the patient had another liver scan five years earlier that showed essentially the same configuration of the liver. Such a configuration of the liver, without or with disease process, has been described as scintigraphic appearance of Riedel's lobe of the liver (Lipchik E.O., Schwartz S.I.: Angiographic and scintillographic identification of Riedel's lobe of the liver. *Radiology* 88:48, 1967).

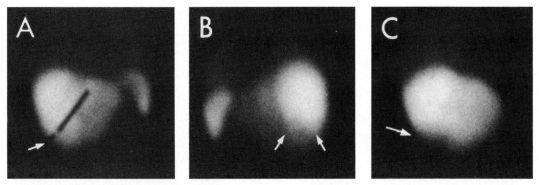

Case 6–9.—Absent Inferior Tip of the Right Lobe of the Liver

Anterior **(A)**, posterior **(B)**, and right lateral **(C)** views of a liver and spleen scan obtained using technetium Tc-99m sulfur colloid show absent inferior tip of the liver *(arrows)*.

Such a finding has been described as an infrequent variant in 1%–2% of normal livers (McAfee J.G., Ause R.G., Wagner H.N.: Diagnostic value of scintillation scanning of the liver. *Arch Intern. Med.* 116:95, 1965).

Such absence of the inferior tip most likely is due to the renal impression-extrinsic compression of the liver in individuals with thin or small frames.

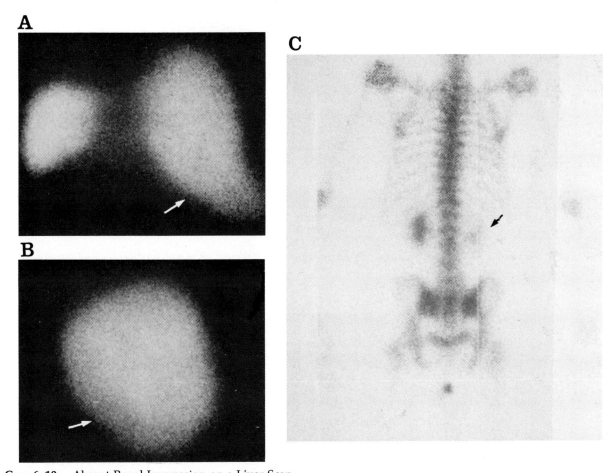

Case 6–10.—Absent Renal Impression on a Liver Scan

Posterior **(A)** and right lateral **(B)** views of a liver scan obtained using technetium Tc-99m sulfur colloid on a 51-year-old woman who had bilateral breast carcinoma show no evidence of renal impression in the posterior right lobe of the liver *(arrow)*.

The renal impression in the posterior liver may disappear after a right nephrectomy. In this patient, however, the right kidney is present as shown on a posterior bone image **(C,** *arrow)*. She had undergone salpingo-oophorectomy five years earlier, and the right kidney became slightly ptotic.

The finding is another example that demonstrates the high pliability of the liver that readily changes its configuration and location with changes in surroundings and gravitational status.

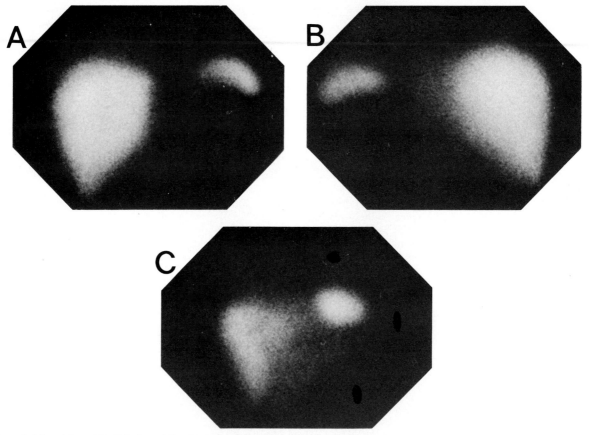

Case 6–11.—Absent Left Lobe of the Liver and Semilunar Spleen

Liver and spleen scan was obtained using technetium Tc-99m sulfur colloid, 4 mCi, on a 83-year-old woman with elevated liver enzyme values. The anterior **(A)** and posterior **(B)** images show normal radionuclide distribution in the liver. However, the left lobe of the liver is absent. Congenital agenesis of the left lobe is known to be rare, with an incidence of 1 in 19,000 cases (Merrill G.G.: Complete absence of the left lobe of the liver. *Arch. Pathol.* 42:232, 1946).

The spleen is semilunar and unusually small, though its configuration appears essentially normal on the left lateral view **(C)**.

The patient was found to have mild congestive heart failure, and results of upper gastrointestinal studies were all normal.

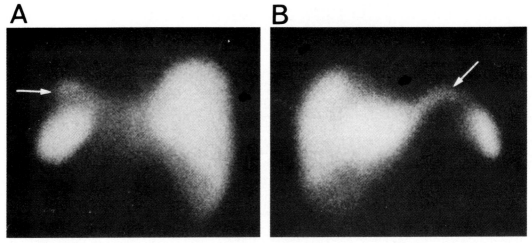

Case 6–12.—"Tongue" of the Left Lobe of the Liver Extended Posteriorly

Posterior **(A)** and left anterior oblique **(B)** views of a liver and spleen scan obtained on a 43-year-old woman with breast carcinoma show stretched-out "tongue" of the left lobe of the liver *(arrow)*. Such posteriorly stretched-out tongue of the liver often causes a scan finding that mimics a splenic lesion on the posterior image (Ryo U.Y.: An artifact that simulates an infarction on a posterior view spleen scan. *J. Nucl. Med.* 16:99, 1975).

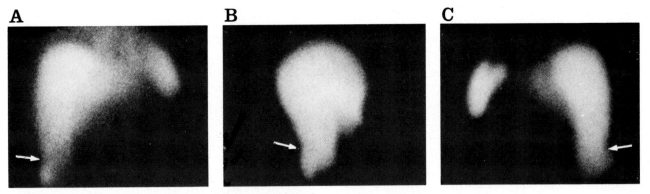

Case 6–13.—Costal Indentation on a Liver and Spleen Scan

Liver and spleen scan, early anterior **(A)** view, right lateral **(B)** and posterior **(C)** views, obtained on a 84-year-old woman with colon carcinoma shows an obvious extrinsic compression at inferior right lobe of the liver, anteriorly and laterally *(arrows)*.

Such impression by the right rib cage is frequently seen on a liver scan of thin patients, and is especially common in elderly women who customarily wear corsets.

The anterior image **(A)** was taken soon after the injection; thus, prominent cardiac blood pool activity is seen.

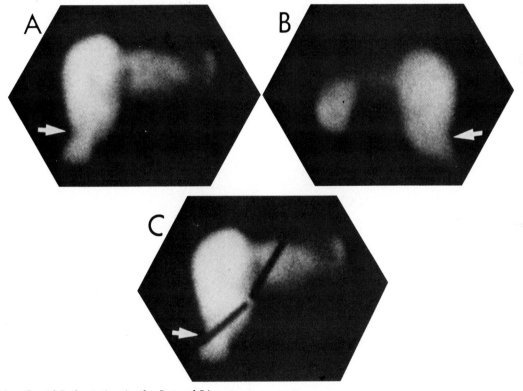

Case 6–14.—Costal Indentation in the Lateral Liver

Anterior **(A)** and posterior **(B)** images of the liver obtained using a 4-mCi dose of technetium Tc-99m sulfur colloid show a prominent defect in the lateral inferior liver *(arrow)*. Such indentation is a common finding in a relatively thin person and in women who customarily use tight corsets. In this case the identation is caused by the right rib cage as shown in the anterior image with right costal marker **(C)**.

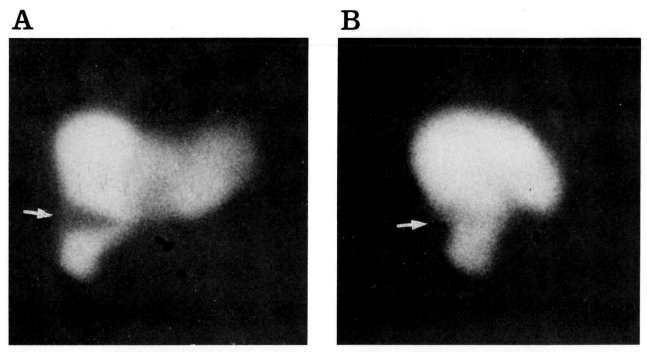

Case 6–15.—Unusually Prominent Costal Indentation on a Liver Scan; An Attenuation Artifact Due to Metallic Girdle

Anterior **(A)** and right lateral **(B)** views of a liver scan obtained using technetium Tc-99m sulfur colloid on a 60-year-old woman show abnormally prominent costal indentation in the lateral inferior liver *(arrow)*. The shape is extremely unusual as a costal indentation because of the razor-edge and the degree and size of the defect.

An examination of the patient revealed a metallic girdle she had been wearing for several years since she had fractured her right arm. The girdle was used to hold the fractured arm.

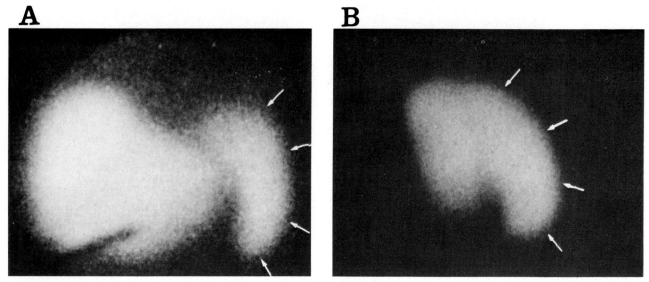

Case 6–16.—Prominent Left Lobe of the Liver on a Right Lateral View Liver Scan Due to Superimposition of the Spleen Image

Right lateral view liver scan obtained with technetium Tc-99m sulfur colloid **(B)** shows an unusually prominent left lobe of the liver *(arrows)*.

The anterior image **(A)**, however, shows that a superimposed image of the enlarged spleen *(arrows)* caused the falsely prominent left lobe.

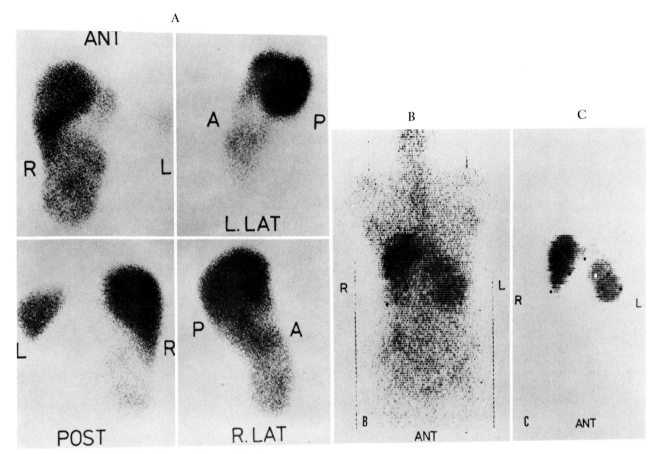

Case 6–17.—Mobile Accessory Lobe of the Liver

Liver and spleen scan was obtained on a 21-year-old woman with suspected brucellosis using a 4-mCi dose of technetium Tc-99m sulfur colloid **(A).** The scan finding was thought to represent a large Riedel's lobe.

However, a gallium scan with a 2.5 mCi dose obtained in order to evaluate the cause of unresolving fever **(B)** showed a large gallium-positive mass in the left hypochondrium, and the "large Riedel's lobe" was no longer present. Repeated liver and spleen images **(C)** were obtained with technetium Tc-99m sulfur colloid immediately after the gallium scan in the same position (supine). The repeated image showed the mass in the left hypochondrium to be a mobile liver lobe. Additional imaging study with technetium Tc-99m-labeled, denatured autologous red blood cells confirmed that the mobile mass was not the spleen but a liver lobe.

(Courtesy of Bingham J.B., Maisey M.N. [Guy's Hospital, London]: Unusual scintigraphic appearances of a mobile accessory lobe of the liver. *J. Nucl. Med.* 19:1235, 1978.)

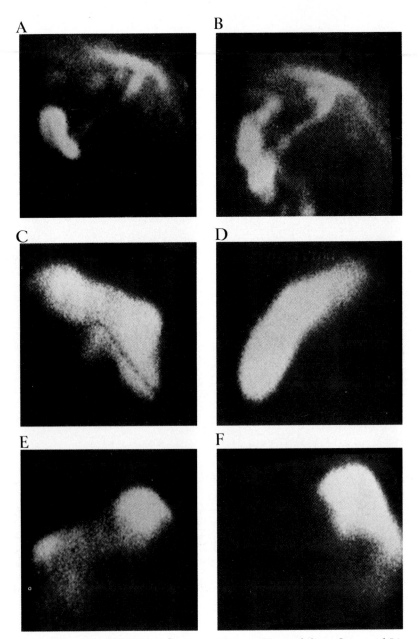

Case 6–18.—Asplenia Syndrome With Situs Inversus Seen on Hepatobiliary Scan and Liver and Spleen Scan

Hepatobiliary scan was performed on a 26-year-old woman with sudden onset of nausea, pain, and mass in the upper abdomen. The images obtained after an intravenous dose of technetium Tc 99m lidofenin-o-dimethyl iminodiacetic acid showed left-sided liver **(A** and **B).** Biliary tracts and excretion of the radionuclide into the intestine were observed.

To confirm the anomalous position of the liver, a liver and spleen scan was obtained using technetium Tc-99m sulfur colloid. The anterior **(C),** left lateral **(D),** posterior **(E),** and right lateral **(F)** views confirmed the position of the liver, which occupied the left upper quadrant. The spleen was absent. The absence of the spleen was reconfirmed by an observations of Howell-Jolly bodies on a peripheral blood smear. Other anomalies found in this patient included right-sided stomach, duodenum, and small intestine. The ascending colon, cecum, and proximal transverse colon were on the left. However, the heart and major vessels were in normal positions. Summary of the findings led to the diagnosis of asplenia syndrome of the partial visceral situs inversus type.

(Courtesy of Hauser G.J., Silverman C. [Soroka Medical Center, Beer-Sheva, Israel]: Incidental discovery of asplenia syndrome, with situs inversus and a normal heart by radionuclide biliary imaging: A case report. *Clin. Nucl. Med.* 7:543, 1982.)

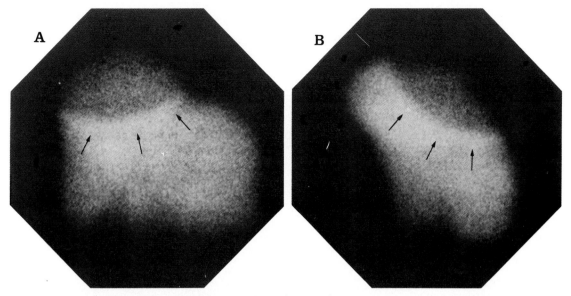

Case 6–19.—"Hot Stripe Sign" on a Liver Scan; A Typical Example

Anterior **(A)** and right lateral views of a liver scan obtained on a 34-year-old woman, using technetium Tc-99m sulfur colloid show curvilinear hot line along with inferior border of the photon-deficient area *(arrows)* at the anterior dome of the liver. The finding is a typical example of the photon attenuation by the breast and "hot stripe" formed by the small-angle scattering of photons (Ryo U.Y., Wilczak D.J., Kim I. et al.: A scan artifact caused by a band of scattered photons. *Radiology* 146:840, 1983).

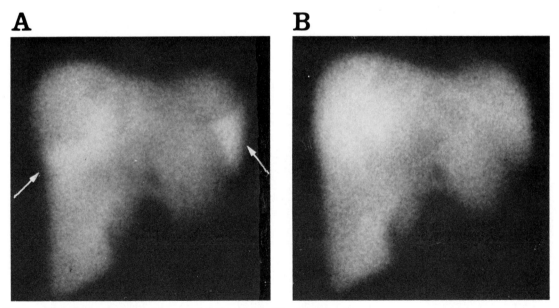

Case 6–20.—"Hot Stripe" on the Liver and Spleen on a Liver-Spleen Scan

Anterior image of the liver and spleen obtained using technetium Tc-99m sulfur colloid shows "hot stripes" over the right lobe of the liver as well as over the lower half of the spleen (**A,** *arrows*).

The "hot stripes" disappeared on a repeated anterior image obtained while the both right and left breast were held cephalad **(B).**

Thus, the "hot stripe" may also appear over the anterior spleen image when there is splenomegaly and when enough photons from the spleen are scattered through the left breast.

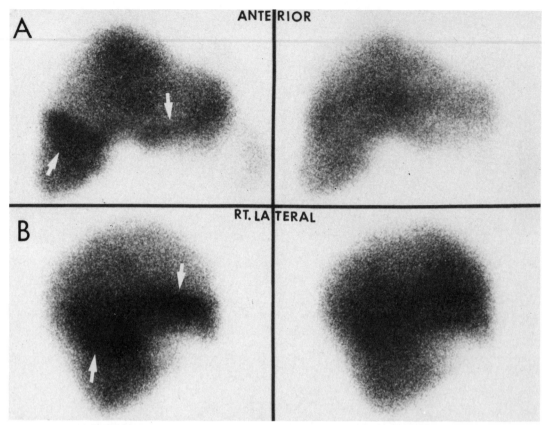

Case 6–21.—"Hot Stripe" on a Liver Scan That May Cause False Positive Scan Interpretation

Liver scan **(I)**, anterior **(A)** and right lateral **(B)** views, obtained using technetium Tc-99m sulfur colloid on a 68-year-old woman who was receiving chemotherapy for colon carcinoma, shows a markedly inhomogeneous uptake with areas of increased *(arrows)* and decreased uptake. The finding may lead to a false interpretation of Budd-Chiari syndrome or liver cirrhosis.

Repeated views obtained while the right breast was held cephalad show no areas with relatively increased uptake, demonstrating another example of "hot stripe" caused by a band of photons scattered through the breast tissue.

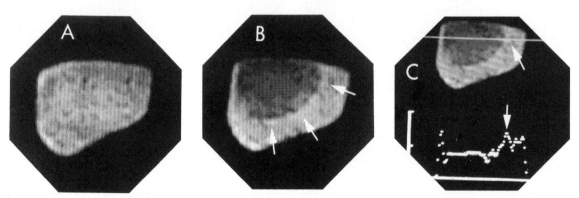

Case 6–22.—Demonstration of the Small-angle Scattering of Photons Causing the "Hot Stripe" on the Liver Scan

A, liver phantom made of short-grain rice in a vinyl bag mixed with water and a 1-mCi dose of technetium Tc-99m sulfur colloid.

B, breast phantom, smaller vinyl bag with rice and water without radionuclide, was placed over the liver phantom, simulating a breast attenuation of photons from the liver. The scan of two phantoms shows a large crescent defect that is surrounded by a rim of accentuated radioactivity *(arrows)*, reproducing the "hot stripe" on a liver scan.

C, transaxial slice of the phantom image and the profile of the radioactivity distribution show the rim activity—"hot stripe"—to be actual collection of the photons; thus, the phantom study proves that the "hot stripe" on a liver scan is formed by a band of scattered photons.

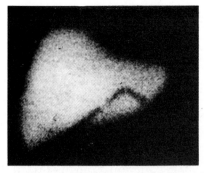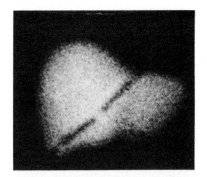

Case 6–23.—Position and Configuration of the Liver Change as the Position of the Patient Changes

A, example of anterior liver image obtained with technetium Tc-99m sulfur colloid on a 35-year-old man showing essentially normal size and configuration of the liver.

B, repeated anterior liver image on the same patient obtained at upright position. When the position of the patient was changed from supine **(A)** to upright **(B)**, the vertical span of the liver increased; in particular, the left lobe became larger and the quadrate lobe became apparent.

The configuration of the liver changes so much at different positions that a follow-up scan may appear as a scan of a different patient or may cause a false interpretation of hepatomegaly, congestion, etc.

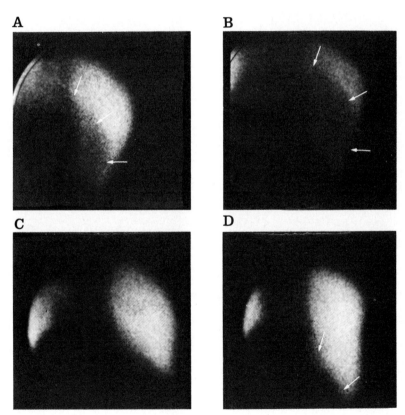

Case 6–24.—Effect of Positional Changes on the Renal Impression of the Posterior Liver

Two example cases of renal impression seen on a posterior liver scan, obtained using technetium Tc-99m sulfur colloid:

Case 1: Posterior liver scan taken at supine position shows normal renal impression (**A,** *arrow*). Same posterior view taken at upright position shows abnormally prominent renal impression (**B,** *arrows*).

Case 2: Posterior liver scan taken at supine position shows no obvious renal impression **(C).** Same posterior view taken at upright position shows vertical position of the liver and identifiable renal impression at the inferior border (**D,** *arrows*).

On a posterior liver scan, height of the liver increases, and the renal impression becomes significantly larger when the image is taken at an upright, standing position.

When an unusually prominent renal impression is noted on a posterior liver scan, position of the patient at the time of imaging should be checked.

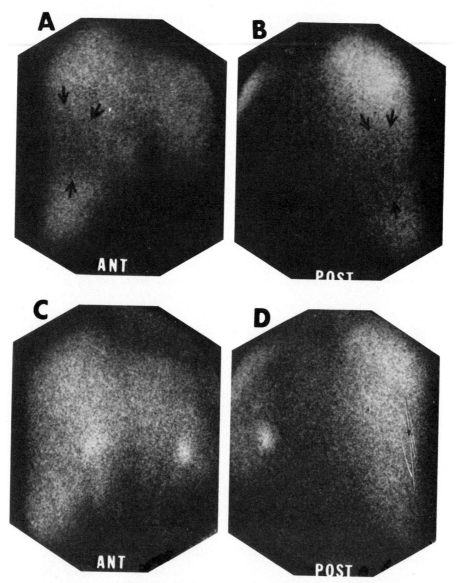

Case 6–25.—Prominent Renal Impression Causing Defects on Liver Scan, on the Anterior View as Well as the Posterior View; Example Case 1

Liver scan, obtained on a 32-year-old man, using technetium Tc-99m sulfur colloid, shows a large, ill-defined defect seen on the anterior image (**A**, *arrows*). Posterior view scan shows prominent renal impression that extends to the lateral margin of the right lobe (**B**, *arrows*). Repeat anterior (**C**) and posterior (**D**) views obtained ten minutes after an intravenous injection of technetium Tc-99m pentetic acid show completed filling of the "defects" by the renal activity. Radioactivity in the renal pelvis appears more pronounced on the anterior view (**C**).

Such prominent renal impression on the liver image is frequently seen in thin individuals and may cause false positive interpretations of a liver scan. (Ryo U.Y., Siddiqui A., Yum H.Y., et al.: Focal defect due to renal impression in anterior liver imaging. *Clin. Nucl. Med.* 1:64, 1976.)

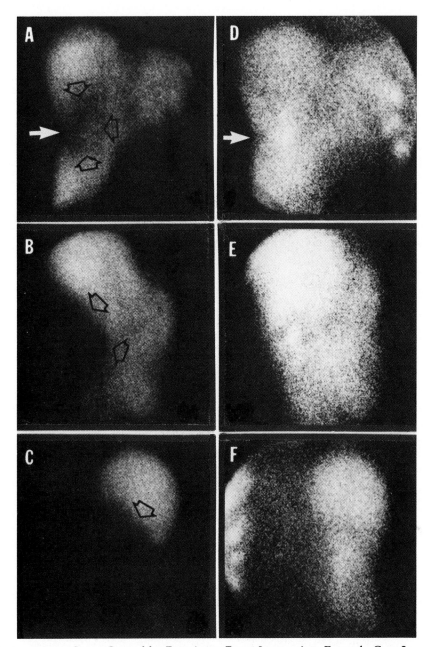

Case 6–26.—Defects on Liver Scans Caused by Prominent Renal Impression; Example Case 2

Liver scan obtained using technetium Tc-99m sulfur colloid on a 66-year-old woman with colon carcinoma, at upright position shows large defect with irregular border on the anterior image *(open arrows)*. Anterior image also shows a prominent costal indentation *(solid arrow)*. Right lateral view **(B)** and posterior view **(C)** show unusually prominent renal impression *(open arrows)*.

Repeated anterior **(D)**, right lateral **(E)**, and posterior views **(F)** obtained ten minutes after an injection of technetium Tc-99m pentetic acid show the renal activity filling in the "defects" and renal impression.

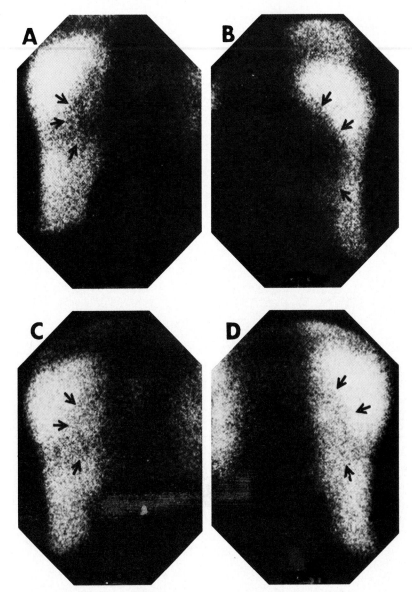

Case 6–27.—Prominent Renal Impression Causing Defects in Anterior-medial Liver on a Liver Scan

Liver scan was obtained using technetium Tc-99m sulfur colloid on a 43-year-old woman with elevated liver enzymes.

The anterior view **(A)** shows a typical Riedel's lobe (Lipchik E.O., Schwartz S.I.: Angiographic and scintillographic identification of Riedel's lobe of the liver. *Radiology* 88:48, 1967) and a large defect in the anterior-medial liver *(arrows)*. The posterior view **(B)** shows prominent renal impression.

Repeated anterior **(C)** and posterior **(D)** liver scan views obtained after an intravenous dose of technetium Tc-99m pentetic acid show a complete filling of the defect by the renal activity *(arrows)*.

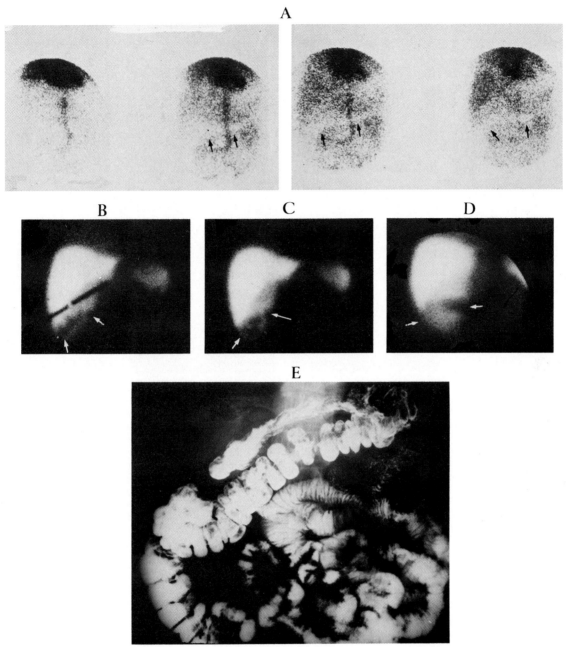

Case 6–28.—Barium in the Colon Causing Artifactitious Defect in the Anterior Liver on a Liver and Spleen Scan

Liver flow study obtained with an intravenous injection of technetium Tc-99m sulfur colloid shows a curvilinear photon-deficient area in the abdomen (**A,** *arrows*). An anterior liver image with right costal marker (**B**) taken at supine position shows a linear defect in the inferior liver *(arrows)*. The shape and location of the defect changed on a repeated anterior (**C**) and right anterior oblique (**D**) views taken at upright position *(arrows)*. The linear defect was an effect of photon attenuation by barium in the hepatic flexure of the colon (**E**).

The haustral marking could be retrospectively recognized in the attenuation defect (**B** and **C**).

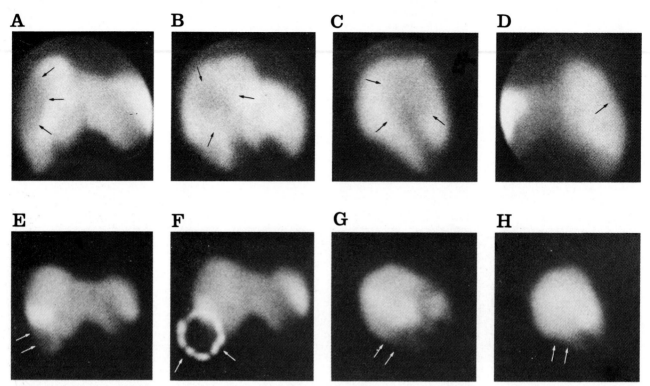

Case 6–29.—Large Defect Demonstrated on a Liver Scan Caused by a Thoracic Wall Cyst; Another Example of Artifactitious Liver Defect

Liver scan, anterior **(A)**, right anterior oblique **(B)**, right lateral **(C)**, and posterior **(D)** views, was obtained on a 46-year-old woman with a large thoracic wall cyst using technetium Tc-99m sulfur colloid, at upright position of the patient.

The scan shows a large defect with a smooth border in the liver *(arrows)*. Ultrasonography revealed that the large defect represented impression of thoracic wall cyst on the liver. A follow-up scan was obtained three years later on the same patient at supine position. The thoracic wall cyst had been reduced in size after aspirations.

Anterior view **(E)**, anterior view with marker over the cyst **(F)**, right oblique view **(G)**, and right lateral view **(H)** show a "compression defect" in the inferior lateral liver, corresponding to thoracic wall cyst *(arrows)*.

Without a direct examination of the patient, the liver scan of this patient might have been falsely interpreted as showing intrahepatic mass lesion.

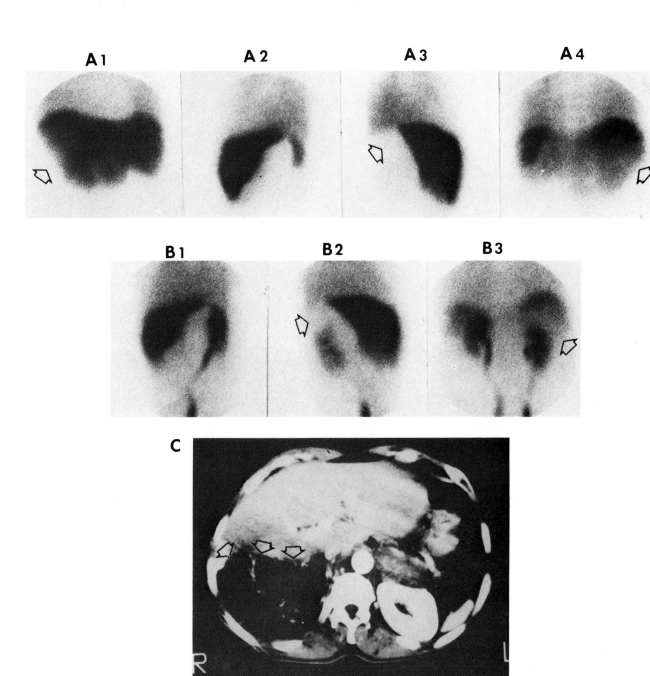

Case 6–30.—Pseudolesion of the Liver; A Large Defect in the Right Lobe of the Liver Caused by Displaced Colon

Liver and spleen scan taken 15 minutes after an intravenous injection of technetium Tc-99m sulfur colloid.

Anterior **(A1),** left lateral **(A2),** right lateral **(A3),** and posterior **(A4)** views show a large right lobe defect *(open arrow).* The right lateral view **(A3)** suggests that there is right renal or suprarenal mass causing the liver defect. Therefore, combined liver-kidney images were subsequently obtained after an additional injection of 10-mCi dose of technetium Tc-99m pentetic acid. The combined image, left lateral **(B1),** right lateral **(B2),** and posterior **(B3)** views, show normal kidneys. There was, however, abnormal separation between the liver and the right kidney **(B2** and **B3,** *arrows).*

Computed tomography of the abdomen with contrast medium infusion **(C)** revealed that there was displaced colon behind the right lobe of the liver, causing a severe deformation of the liver.

(Comment: this is one of many cases of pseudolesion of the liver caused by extrinsic compression, demonstrating again the pliability of the liver. It is, however, very unusual to see such deformation of the liver caused by the large intestine. In a patient with megacolon or with chronic, severe constipation, possible liver deformity due to hepatic flexure of the colon should be considered.)

(Courtesy of Hussein M. Abdel-Dayem, M.D., Professor, Department of Radiology and Nuclear Medicine, Faculty of Medicine, Kuwait University, Safat, Kuwait.)

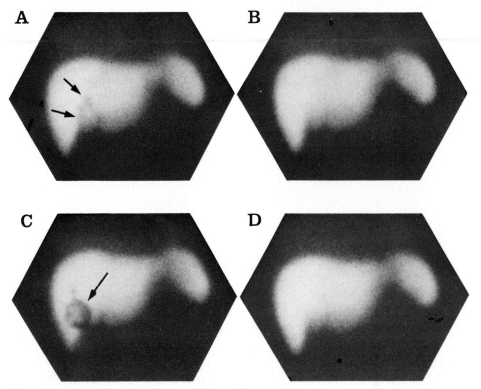

Case 6–31.—Attenuation Artifacts on a Liver and Spleen Scan

Anterior images of liver and spleen scan show irregular, linear defect **(A)** and a round defect **(C)** in the anterior right lobe of the liver *(arrows)* that disappeared when repeated images were taken after a keychain **(B)** and a pocket watch **(D),** respectively, were removed.

Such an attenuation artifact owing to metallic objects in a pocket is a frequent artifact noted on radionuclide images, particularly prevalent on scans of outpatients. The technologist should always remember to ask patients to remove metallic objects from the imaging field.

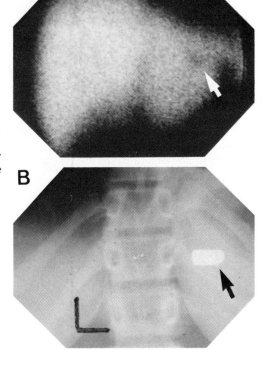

Case 6–32.—Silent Bullet Embedded in the Liver

Anterior liver image **(A)** obtained using technetium Tc-99m sulfur colloid on a 24-year-old man with suspected hepatitis shows a small, space-occupying lesion in the left lobe *(white arrow)*. His plain abdominal radiograph **(B)** showed a bullet in the left lobe of the liver *(black arrow)* corresponding to the defect seen on the liver image. The defect seen on the liver image is not sharply defined because the metal piece is surrounded by normally functioning Kupffer cells that take up the radionuclides. This finding contrasts with the sharp attenuation caused by metallic leads attached on the skin.

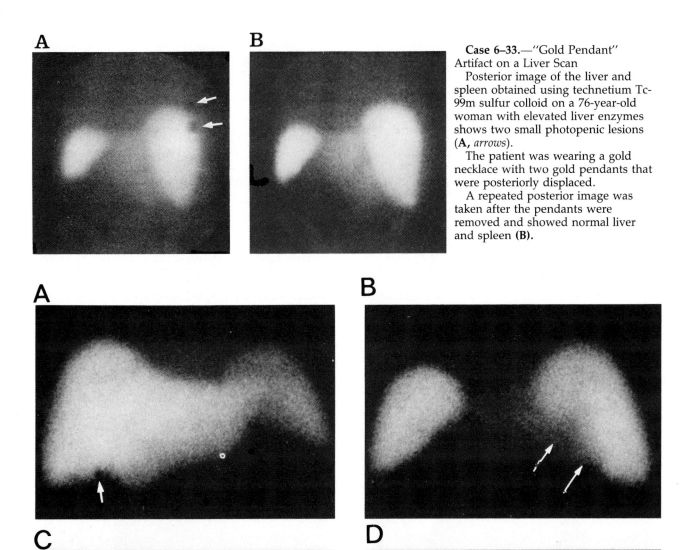

A **B**

Case 6–33.—"Gold Pendant" Artifact on a Liver Scan

Posterior image of the liver and spleen obtained using technetium Tc-99m sulfur colloid on a 76-year-old woman with elevated liver enzymes shows two small photopenic lesions (**A,** *arrows*).

The patient was wearing a gold necklace with two gold pendants that were posteriorly displaced.

A repeated posterior image was taken after the pendants were removed and showed normal liver and spleen (**B**).

Case 6–34.—Indistinct Renal Impression and Monitor Lead Artifact on a Liver and Spleen Scan

Liver and spleen scan was obtained on a 71-year-old man with elevated liver enzymes values, using a 6-mCi dose of technetium Tc-99m sulfur colloid.

The anterior image (**A**) shows a discrete, small defect in the inferior edge of the right lobe *(arrow)*. The defect, however, moved to the inferior left lobe on a right oblique image (**C,** *arrow*).

The artifactitious lesions, attenuation by a lead of a cardiac monitor, is one of the most common artifacts that appears on radionuclide images. The posterior image (**B**) shows indistinct renal impression *(arrows)*.

Location of normal right kidney is lower than usual position in this patient; thus, renal impression is not apparent on the posterior view (**B**) and the right lateral view (**D**).

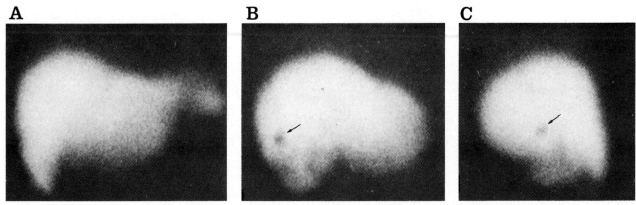

Case 6–35.—Another Example of a Bullet Artifact on a Liver Scan

Liver scan, anterior **(A),** right anterior oblique **(B),** and right lateral **(C)** views, obtained using technetium Tc-99m sulfur colloid on a 60-year-old woman with breast carcinoma shows a small photon-deficient area in the right posterior liver *(arrow).*

The patient had a gunshot wound 20 years ago and carries the silent bullet in the right posterior liver.

Metastatic tumor in the bullet size probably would not be demonstrated on the scan as clearly as the bullet.

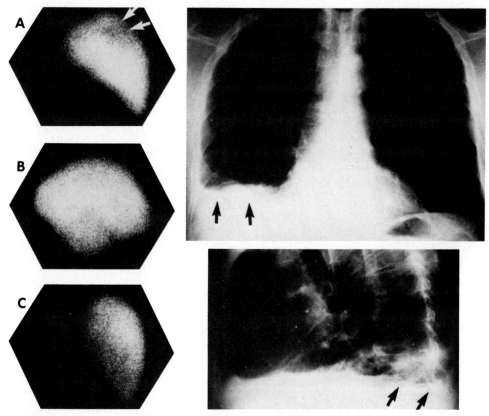

Case 6–36.—Artifactitious Lesion on a Liver Scan Caused by an Infiltrate in the Right Lung Base

Liver scan was obtained using technetium Tc-99m sulfur colloid on a 62-year-old woman with a chief complaint of weight loss and poor appetite. The scan, posterior view **(A),** shows a large, wedge-shaped defect in the posterior dome *(arrows).* The right lateral view **(B),** however, shows no abnormality in the dome. A repeated posterior view taken at upright position **(C)** does not show the lesion that appeared on the initial posterior view taken at supine position.

Chest radiographs, frontal and lateral views, show a large infiltration in the posterior base of the right lung *(black arrows).* This lung infiltration-attenuated photon flux from the dome of the liver caused the artifactitious defect that appeared on the initial posterior view liver scan.

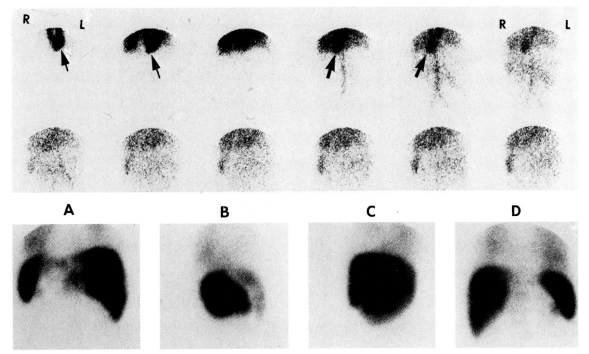

Case 6–37.—Complete Situs Inversus Demonstrated on a Liver-Spleen Study With Technetium Tc-99m Sulfur Colloid

Liver flow study was obtained after a bolus injection of technetium Tc-99m sulfur colloid **(top row)**. The study showed initial filling of left-sided ventricle *(thin arrow)* and later filling of right-sided ventricle *(thick arrow),* indicating that this patient has dextrocardia.

The liver and spleen scan, **A,** anterior view; **B,** right lateral view; **C,** left lateral view; **D,** posterior view, shows the position of the liver and the spleen to be completely reversed: situs inversus.

(Courtesy of Hussein M. Abdel-Dayem, M.D., Professor of Nuclear Medicine, Department of Radiology and Nuclear Medicine, Faculty of Medicine, Kuwait University, Safat, Kuwait.)

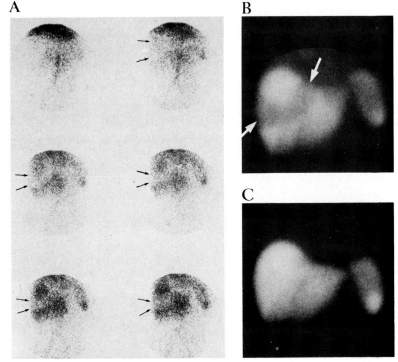

Case 6–38.—Photon Attenuation by Breast Prosthesis on Anterior Liver Flow and Static Images

Dynamic flow images of the liver **(A)** obtained using a bolus injection of technetium Tc-99m sulfur colloid on a 34-year-old woman with breast carcinoma shows a large area of decreased flow in the liver *(arrows).* Anterior static image of the liver **(B)** again demonstrated the large circular area with diminished uptake *(arrows).* The patient was wearing a breast prosthesis.

A repeated anterior image without the breast prosthesis **(C)** shows normal distribution of radionuclide in the liver.

(Comment: this case again demonstrates the importance of direct examination of the patient in order to evaluate properly the findings on the medical images.)

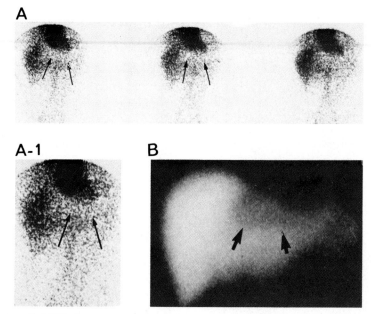

Case 6–39.—Pseudopericardial Effusion

Liver flow study and scan obtained on a 27-year-old woman with Hodgkin's lymphoma using technetium Tc-99m sulfur colloid.

A and **A-1,** the liver flow study shows photopenic region surrounding (?) the ventricular activity. The findings may suggest massive pericardial effusion *(thin arrows)*.

B, the static liver scan shows a rectangular defect, a change from radiation therapy, in the superior left lobe of the liver *(thick arrows)*. This portion of the superior left lobe was included in the field of radiation therapy given to the mediastinum for biopsy-proved lymphoma.

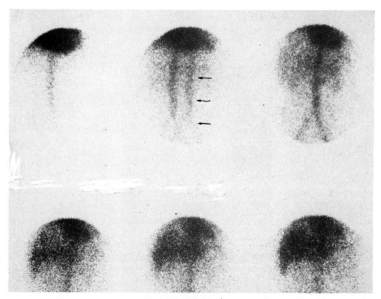

Case 6–40.—Double Abdominal Aorta on Dynamic Hepatic Flow Images; A Motion Artifact

Dynamic hepatic flow image obtained at frame rate of every two seconds after a bolus injection of technetium Tc-99m sulfur colloid shows a double abdominal aorta that appeared only on one frame *(arrows)*.

The technologist who recognized the off-center position of the patient on the first flow image quickly moved the camera, causing the double aorta on the second frame, a motion artifact.

A

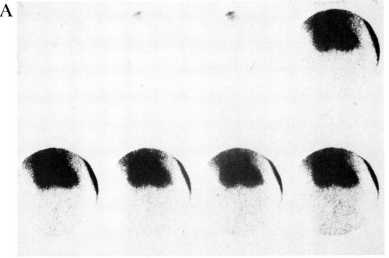

B

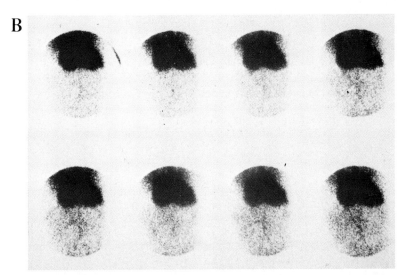

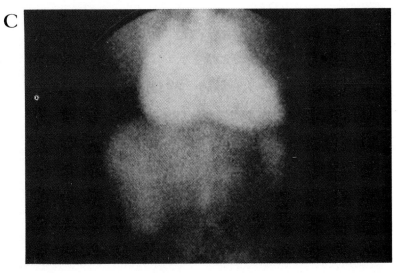

C

Case 6–41.—Suboptimum Hepatic Flow Study Due to Severe Congestive Heart Failure

Hepatic flow study was performed as a part of the liver scan using technetium Tc-99m sulfur colloid on a 49-year-old woman with a childhood history of rheumatic heart disease and triple valve replacements. The dynamic images obtained at rate of five seconds per frame **(A** and **B)** show persistent activity in the heart and hepatic flow was barely recognized in later frames, 60 seconds after the bolus injection.

The blood pool image taken five minutes after the injection **(C)** shows massive cardiomegaly and persistence of radioactivity in the heart and in the major vessels; an example of severe congestive heart failure causing unusual retention of radioactive colloid in the right and left cardiac chambers. The flow of the radioactivity, the "radioactivity output" from the heart, is too low to produce an effective hepatic flow images.

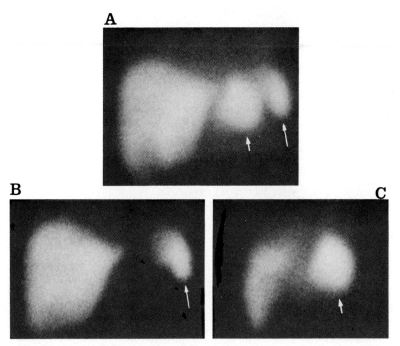

Case 6–42.—Example of Double Spleen (?); Technical Artifact

Left anterior oblique image **(A)** of liver and spleen scan obtained using technetium Tc-99m sulfur colloid shows a double spleen *(arrows)*.

Repeated anterior oblique **(B)** and left lateral **(C)** views show normal, single spleen.

The image **A** was a double exposure, the superimposition of the left anterior oblique and left lateral views, a technical artifact.

Case 6–43.—Extended Left Lobe of the Liver Mimics Image of the Spleen on a Liver and Spleen Scan

Liver and spleen scan obtained on a 30-year-old woman with sickle cell disease shows a small spleen (?, *thin arrow*) on anterior **(A)** and posterior **(B)** images. However, the spleen was not detected on the left lateral view **(C,** *thick arrow).*

A spleen scan with technetium Tc-99m-labeled red blood cells, left lateral view **(D),** failed to demonstrate the spleen *(thick arrow).*

The patient had "autosplenectomy" due to sickle cell disease, and the left lobe of the liver extended into the splenic bed.

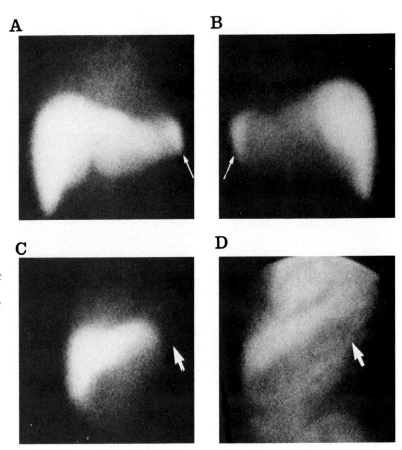

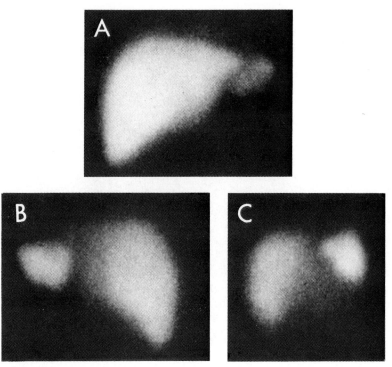

Case 6–44.—Rotation of the Spleen

Liver and spleen scan obtained with technetium Tc-99m sulfur colloid shows medially displaced spleen on the anterior view **(A)**. The posterior **(B)** and left lateral view **(C)** shows that the spleen is 180° rotated from the usual position. The uniform, normal uptake by the spleen indicates normal blood flow.

Such rotation or malposition of the spleen is not an uncommon normal variant.

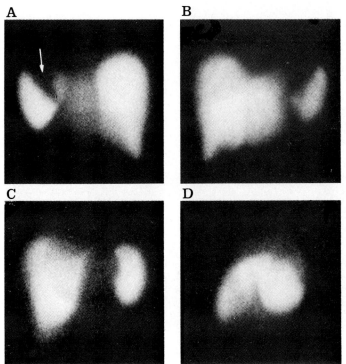

Case 6–45.—"Upside Down" Spleen on a Liver and Spleen Scan

Liver and spleen scan was obtained using technetium Tc-99m sulfur colloid on a 49-year-old woman who was involved in an auto accident.

A posterior view **(A)** shows a triangular "defect" in the superior spleen *(arrow)*. Anterior view **(B)** shows superiorly faced hilum of the spleen. Left anterior oblique **(C)** and left lateral **(D)** views show essentially normal spleen.

The patient had previous liver and spleen scan which showed essentially the same configuration of the spleen. The appearance of the "defect" on posterior view is an artifactitious lesion caused by the margin of the left lobe of the liver and the posterior border of the spleen (Ryo U.Y.: An artifact that simulates an infarction on a posterior view spleen scan. *J. Nucl. Med.* 16:99, 1975). Such upside down spleen with superior facing hilum is a rare variant (Westcott J.L., Krufky E.L.: The upside-down spleen. *Radiology* 105:517, 1972).

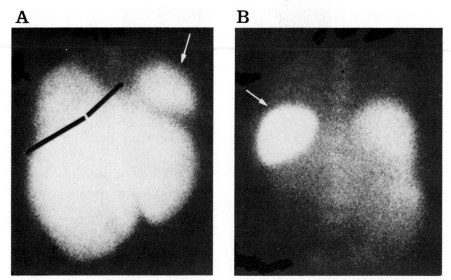

Case 6–46.—Superiorly Displaced Spleen Due to a Massive Hepatomegaly Demonstrated on a Liver-Spleen Scan

Anterior view with right costal marker **(A)** and posterior view **(B)** liver-spleen scan obtained using technetium Tc-99m sulfur colloid on a 68-year-old woman with a long history of congestive heart failure shows a massive hepatomegaly; the liver occupies almost the entire abdomen.

The spleen is located superior to the left lobe of the liver *(arrow)*; very rare variation of location of the spleen that is caused by a massive hepatomegaly.

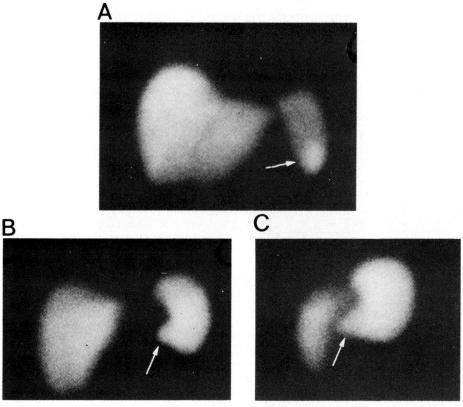

Case 6–47.—Hot Spot in the Spleen

Anterior image of the liver and spleen obtained using technetium Tc-99m sulfur colloid on a 34-year-old woman with breast carcinoma shows a hot spot in the inferior spleen **(A,** *arrow)*.

The left anterior oblique **(B)** and left lateral views **(C)** show a protrusion of inferior spleen anteriorly, causing the "hot spot" in the anterior spleen image. Such "redundant" splenic tissue can also cause a hot spot in a posterior spleen image. (Spencer R.P.: Splenic "hot spot" due to redundant tissue. *Clin. Nucl. Med.* 8:239, 1983.)

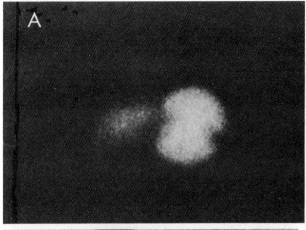

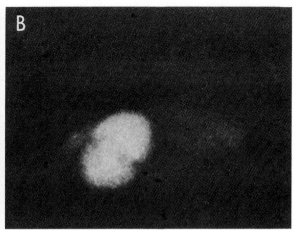

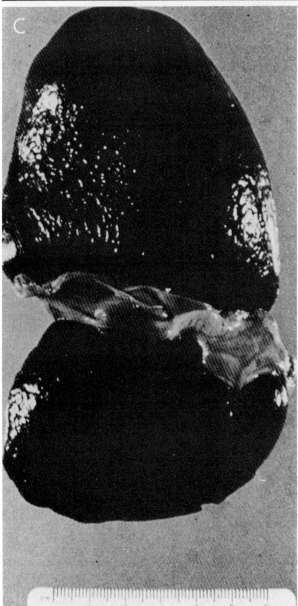

Case 6–48.—Congenital Anomaly of the Spleen; Lobulated Spleen

A and B, liver and spleen scan, anterior (A) and left lateral (B) view, obtained on a 58-year-old man with congestive heart failure and abdominal pain showed a linear defect in the spleen. The finding was thought to represent two notches, presumably congenital, but it mimics a splenic laceration.

C, the patient suffered a cardiac arrest a month later, and the spleen was found at autopsy to be constricted into two lobes.

(Courtesy of D.G. Wilson, L.M. Liberman, [University of Wisconsin Hospital, Madison, Wisconsin]: Unusual splenic band appearance on liver-spleen scan. *Clin. Nucl. Med.* 8:270, 1983.)

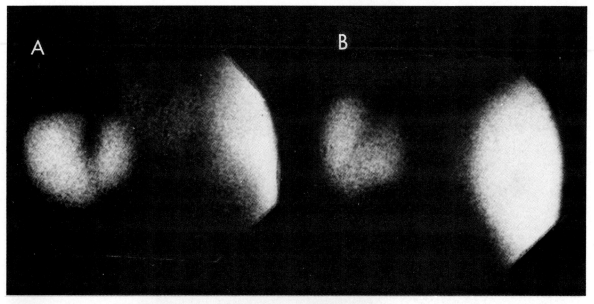

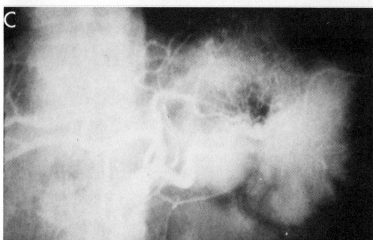

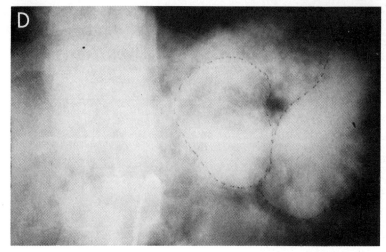

Case 6–49.—Lobulated Spleen; Congenital Anomaly That Simulates Ruptured Spleen.

Spleen scan was obtained using technetium Tc-99m sulfur colloid in a 25-year-old man who complained of left upper quadrant pain after being beaten up by a street gang. The posterior **(A)** and left posterior oblique **(B)** views of the spleen show an abnormal separation of the spleen that is highly suggestive of laceration. Celiac angiogram, early arterial **(C)** and late capillary phases **(D),** show an anomalous spleen—lobulated spleen without laceration.

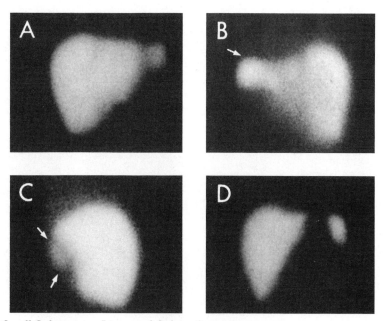

Case 6–50.—Normal, Small Spleen on a Liver and Spleen Scan

Liver and spleen scan was obtained using a 1-mCi dose of technetium Tc-99m sulfur colloid on a 9-year-old girl with Wilms' tumor.

The liver appeared normal on the scan **(A),** 12 cm long, which is within the normal range for a 9-year-old child (Spencer R.P., Banever C.: Growth of the human liver: A preliminary scan study. *J. Nucl. Med.* 11:660, 1970). The spleen was 3.5 cm, which is half the average normal size of the spleen in a 9-year-old child (Spencer R.P., Pearson H.A., Lange R.C.: Human spleen: Scan studies on growth and response to medications. *J. Nucl. Med.* 12:466, 1971), but is at the low end of the normal range. The child had no evidence of hematologic or splenic disease.

An upright right lateral image **(C)** shows an artifactitious liver lesion caused by the image of the spleen *(arrows).* When a right lateral view becomes a slightly posterior oblique projection, the spleen becomes visualized posteriorly, and thus may cause the false appearance of a liver lesion.

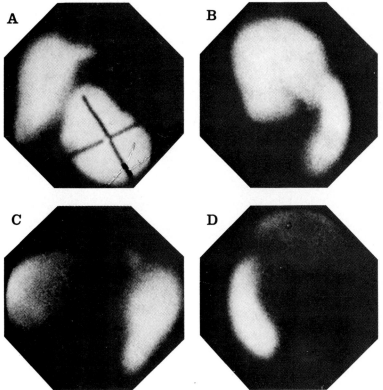

Case 6–51.—"Wandering Spleen" Demonstrated on a Liver and Spleen Scan

Anterior **(A),** right lateral **(B),** left anterior oblique **(C),** and left lateral **(D)** views of liver and spleen scans were obtained using technetium Tc-99m sulfur colloid on a 24-year-old woman with a large abdominal mass.

The anterior view was obtained with lead marker, 10-cm strips, placed over the mass. The mass measured 20 cm, and the uptake of the radiocolloid by the mass indicated that it was the spleen.

The scan findings are consistent with "wandering spleen," which was located in the anterior low abdomen at the time.

Frequent rotation and compression of the splenic vein causes gradual splenomegaly in many cases. Frequently, such wandering spleen suffers tortion of the pedicle. (Abell G.: Wandering spleen with torsion of the pedicle. *Ann. Surg.* 98:722, 1933.)

Case 6–52.—Accessory Spleen

Liver and spleen scan on a 63-year-old woman with colon carcinomas. The anterior **(A)** and left lateral **(B)** views show a small accessory spleen located below the tip of the spleen *(arrow).*

(Comment: the incidence of the accessory spleen is known in the literature as around 11% (Halpert B., Gyorkey F.: Lesions observed in accessory spleen of 311 patients. *Am. J. Clin. Path.* 32:165, 1959). However, the incidence of imaging the accessory spleen on a scan is much lower, because the majority of the accessory spleen is nonfunctional and/or located in the hilar region, too close to the spleen to be visualized as separate tissue.)

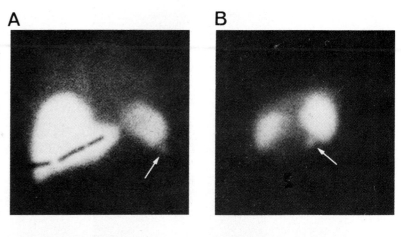

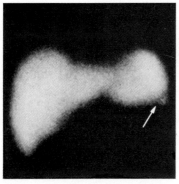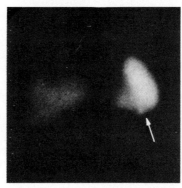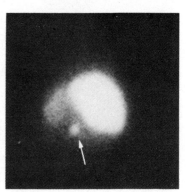

Case 6–53.—Accessory Spleen on a Liver and Spleen Scan; Another Example

Liver and spleen scan, anterior **(A),** left anterior oblique **(B),** and left lateral **(C)** views, obtained using technetium Tc-99m sulfur colloid on a 33-year-old woman with history of hepatitis, shows an accessory spleen near the inferior spleen.

In 80% of cases, the accessory spleen is located at the splenic hilus or in the splenic pedicle (Curtis, G.M., Movitz D.: The surgical significance of the accessory spleen. *Ann. Surg.* 123:276, 1946) and thus is not visualized on a liver and spleen scan.

The accessory spleen detected on a liver and spleen scan with technetium Tc-99m sulfur colloid usually is found at or near the inferior border of the spleen.

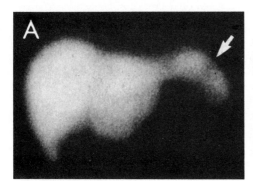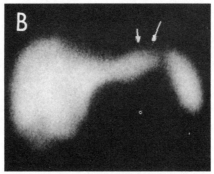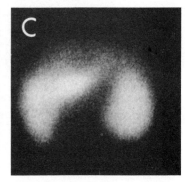

Case 6–54.—"Tongue" of the Liver Causing Artifactitious Defect on a Spleen Image

Liver-spleen scan was obtained on a 61-year-old man with lung carcinoma using technetium Tc-99m sulfur colloid.

A, anterior image showed a linear defect in the anterior spleen *(arrow).*

B, left anterior oblique view showed an elongated left lobe of the liver—a tongue *(small arrows)*—extending to the left upper quadrant.

C, left lateral view showed essentially normal spleen.

The upper part of the spleen in this case is thinner than lower part and more posteriorly positioned. The anterior view, therefore, would have shown lower radioactivity in the upper spleen than in the lower part, but the extended "tongue of the liver" in front of the upper spleen caused an artifactitious defect on the anterior spleen image.

(Comment: such extended "tongue of the liver" is a common finding in a patient who received a splenectomy; however, it is uncommon in the presence of a normal spleen.)

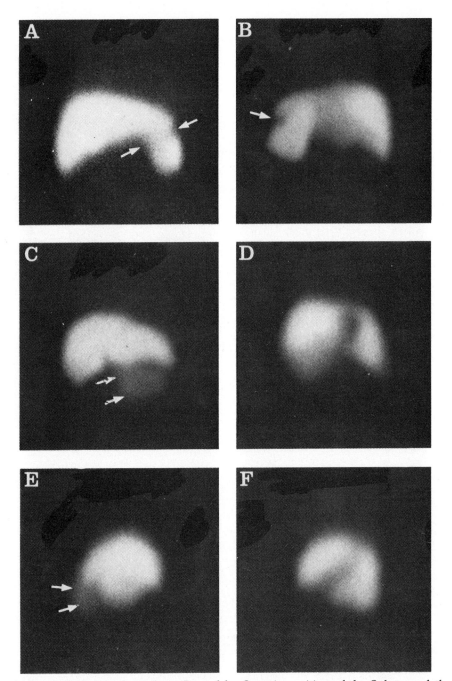

Case 6–55.—Artifactitious Defect in the Spleen Caused by Superimposition of the Spleen and the Liver on a Liver and Spleen Scan

Liver and spleen scan obtained with technetium Tc-99m sulfur colloid on a 20-month-old boy with stage IV neuroblastoma shows a "square spleen," a normal variant. Anterior **(A)** and posterior **(B)** views show a linear defect in the anterior spleen *(arrows)*. However, the spleen is essentially normal, without defect on the left anterior oblique **(D)** and left lateral **(F)** views. Inferior portion of the spleen appears as area of diminished uptake on the right anterior oblique **(C)** and right lateral **(E)** views *(arrows)*. Superimposition of the liver and spleen often cause artifactitious defects in the spleen.

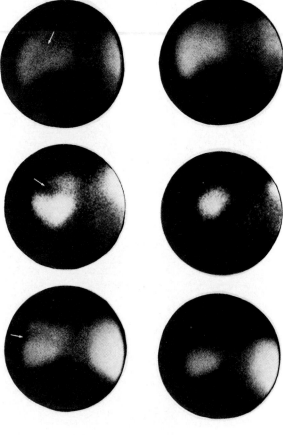

Case 6–56.—Artifact That Simulates Splenic Defects on a Posterior View Spleen Scan

Three examples of posterior spleen scans obtained using technetium Tc-99m sulfur colloid. The initial images **(left row),** all taken at supine position, show wedge-shaped defects *(arrows).*

These defects were no longer present on repeated posterior images taken at upright position **(right row).**

In addition, the spleen appears to be much smaller on the upright scans. Superimposition of the spleen and the left lobe of the liver often forms such artifactitious splenic defects (Ryo U.Y.: An artifact that simulates an infarction on a posterior view spleen scan. *J. Nucl. Med.* 16:99, 1975), and the artifact disappears on the upright view because the liver moves more readily than the spleen with the gravity change. The true image of the spleen is seen on an upright scan, without superimposition of the left lobe of the liver.

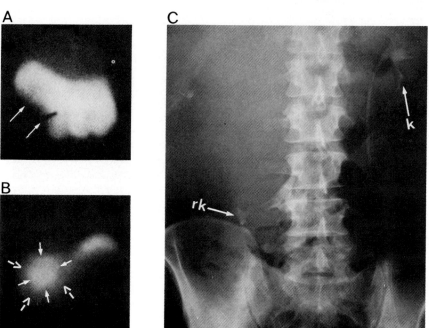

Case 6–57.—Compression Defect in the Right Lobe of the Liver, and "Hidden Spleen" Behind the Left Lobe of the Liver

Liver and spleen scan was obtained on a 59-year-old man with a large right upper quadrant mass. The anterior liver and spleen image **(A)** shows a large defect in the inferior right lobe *(arrows).* The spleen was not visualized on the image. The posterior image **(B)** shows only a small portion of the dome of the liver. The spleen *(small, solid arrows)* is located behind the left lobe of the liver *(open arrows).*

An intravenous pyelographic film **(C)** shows a marked downward displacement of the right kidney *(rk)* by a large soft tissue mass *(k, left kidney).*

A large right adrenal cyst was surgically removed later. The large defect seen in the anterior liver was a compression effect of the adrenal cyst.

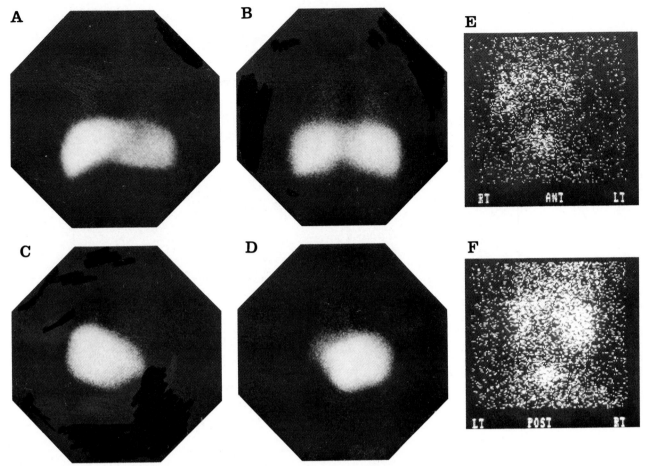

Case 6–58.—Ivemark's Syndrome (Asplenia) Seen on a Liver and Spleen Scan

Liver and spleen scan, anterior **(A),** posterior **(B),** right lateral **(C),** and left lateral **(D)** views, obtained using technetium Tc-99m sulfur colloid on a 2-week-old infant boy shows enlarged left lobe of the liver, and the spleen is not clearly delineated.

Clinically the infant was suspected to have Ivemark's syndrome; therefore, a spleen scan was obtained using Chromium Cr 51-labeled red blood cells (RBCs). Anterior **(E)** and posterior **(F)** digital images over the abdomen shows no evidence of the spleen; thus, asplenia is confirmed.

(Comments: an enlarged left lobe of the liver in the absence of the spleen may be falsely identified as the spleen **(B).** In such cases, a specific spleen scan with technetium Tc-99m-labeled, heat-damaged RBCs is the recommended procedure to confirm presence or absence of the spleen.)

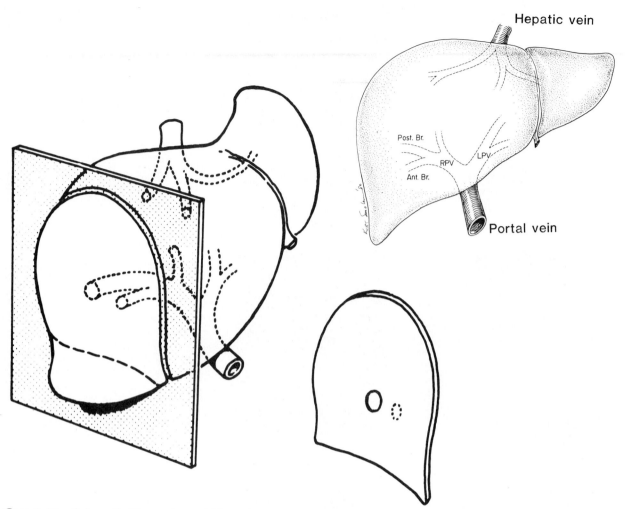

Hepatic vein

Post. Br.

RPV LPV

Ant. Br.

Portal vein

Case 6–59.—Schematic Illustrations of Normal, Intra-hepatic Vascular Structures: Hepatic Vein, Portal Vein and Its Main Branches Shown in Relation to Hepatic Lobes

RPV, right portal vein; LPV, left portal vein. **Post. Br.,** posterior branch; **Ant. Br.,** anterior branch.

Left: scheme showing structural relationship between the anterior and posterior branches of the right portal vein and sagittal slices of emission tomogram.

The normal vascular structure rarely causes defects on planar liver scans. However, intra-hepatic vessels that are 2 cm or larger in diameter may appear as distinct focal defects on emission computed tomograms due to higher sensitivity of the technique (Pettigrew R.I., Witztum K.F., Perkins G.C.: Single photon emission computed tomograms of the liver: Normal vascular intrahepatic structures. *Radiology,* 150:219, 1984).

Understanding of normal intra-hepatic vascular structure, therefore, is very important to avoid false-positive interpretations of emission computed tomography of the liver.

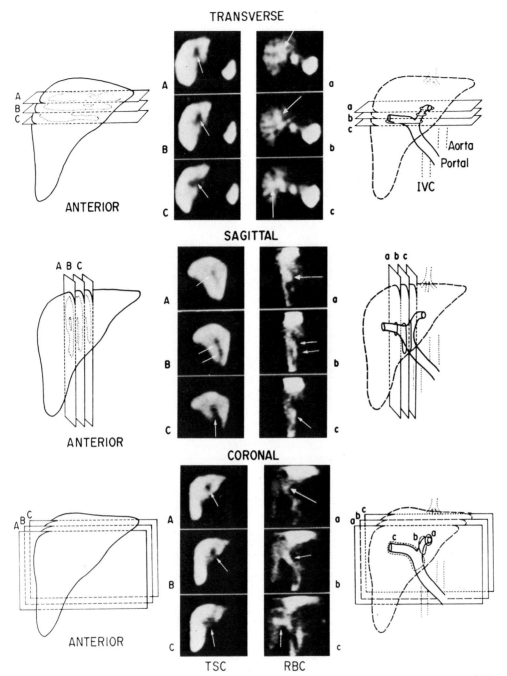

TRANSVERSE

SAGITTAL

CORONAL

TSC   RBC

Case 6–60.—Normal Intrahepatic Vascular Structures on Various Sections of Emission Computed Tomograms, Example Case 1

Transverse, sagittal, and coronal sections of the liver image obtained using Tc-99m sulfur colloid **(TSC)** and with Tc-99m red blood cell **(RBC)** on a patient with enlarged right lobe of the liver but with normal liver functions show defects in various forms that represent portal vein. **Transverse Sections:** large defect seen in slices **A** and **B** of **TSC** image *(arrows)* correspond to the left portal vein as demonstrated on slices **a** and **b** from blood pool image with **RBC** *(arrows)*. The right portal vein caused the large defect which appeared on the slice **C** of **TSC** image *(arrow)*.

Sagittal Sections: the left portal vein **(a,** *arrow)* appears as a small defect on a sagittal slice of **TSC** image **(A,** *arrow)*, while the bifurcation of the right and left portal vein caused linear defect seen on the sagittal slices **B** and **C** *(arrrows)*.

Coronal Sections: anterior slices of the coronal sections of **TSC** images **(A** & **B)** show well-demarcated round defect *(arrow)* that represents the left portal vein as shown on the blood pool images **(a** & **b,** *arrows)*.

The right portal vein and part of the bifurcation caused the large defect shown on the slice **C** *(arrow)* of the **TSC** image.

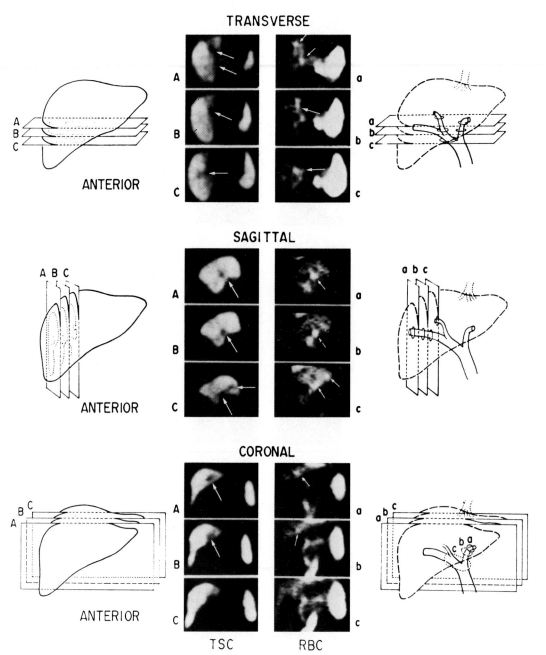

TRANSVERSE

SAGITTAL

CORONAL

TSC RBC

Case 6–61.—Normal Intrahepatic Vascular Structures on Various Sections of Emission Computed Tomograms, Example Case 2

Transverse, sagittal and coronal sections of the liver image obtained using Tc-99m sulfur colloid **(TSC)** on a patient who has a typical triangular liver with normal functions.

Transverse Sections: the left portal vein and the anterior branch of the right portal vein appear as defects on transverse slices (**A** and **B** of **TSC** image [*arrows*]).

Corresponding slices of the blood pool image, **a** and **b**, show the vascular structures *(arrows)*.

Sagittal Sections: sagittal slices of the **TSC** image show round defect in the portal region (**A** & **B**, *arrows*) that correspond to the posterior branch of the right portal vein (**a** & **b**, *arrows*). Both anterior and posterior branches of the right portal vein caused defects in the anterior right lobe as well as a larger defect in the portal region (**C**, *arrows*) on the tomograms.

Coronal Sections: coronal slices of the liver image show defect in the left lobe near to the porta (**A** & **B**, *arrows*) that correspond to the left portal vein (**a** & **b**, *arrows*).

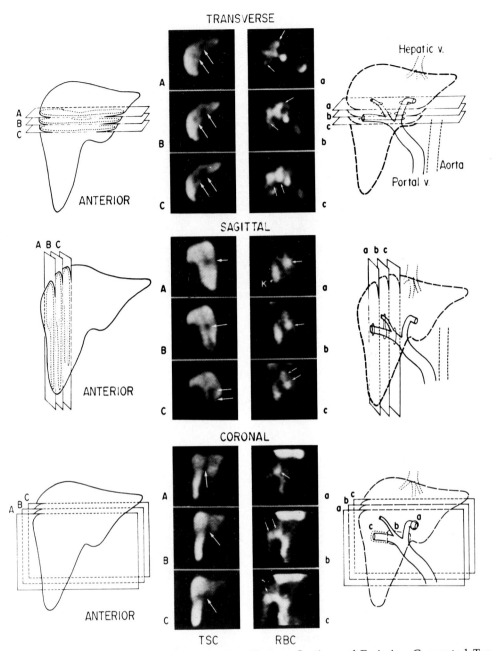

Case 6–62.—Normal Intrahepatic Vascular Structures on Various Sections of Emission Computed Tomograms, Example Case 3

Transverse, sagittal and coronal sections of the liver image obtained on a patient who has "Riedel's lobe" of the liver with normal liver functions show right and left portal vein as defects in Tc-99m sulfur colloid **(TSC)** images and as major vessel on Tc-99m red blood cells **(RBC)** images.

Transverse Sections: slices **A** and **B** of TSC image show larger defect *(arrow)* in the left lobe corresponding to the left portal vein and a smaller defect *(arrow)* in the right lobe corresponding to the anterior branch of the right portal vein. Slice **C** shows a large, elongated defect caused by the bifurcation of the portal vein.

Sagittal Sections: sagittal slices of **TSC** image (**A** and **B**) show well-demarcated round defect *(arrows)* that corresponds to the posterior branch of the right portal vein. The bifurcation caused larger defect on the slice **C.**

Coronal Sections: the coronal slices reveal the Riedel's lobe well. The portal vein, the left branch, right branch and the bifurcation caused defects on slices **A, B,** and **C** *(arrows)*.

SAGITTAL

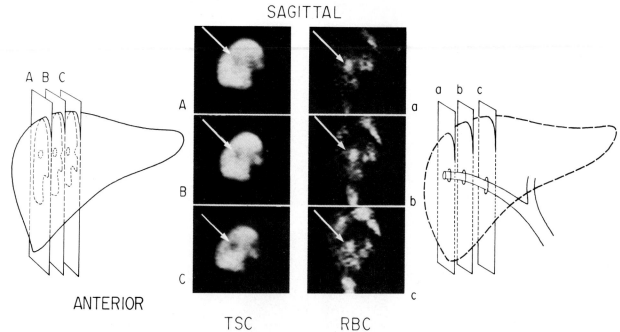

ANTERIOR

TSC   RBC

Case 6–63.—Posterior Branch of the Right Portal Vein Causing a Large "Defect" on Sagittal Sections of the Emission Computed Tomograms of the Liver

The sagittal slices of the right lobe of the liver show fairly large, round defect in the deep liver parenchyma *(arrows).* The defect is not in the usual region of the porta.

The same sagittal slices of the blood pool image of the liver **(RBC)** show that the defects correspond to the posterior branch of the right portal vein *(arrow).*

TRANSVERSE

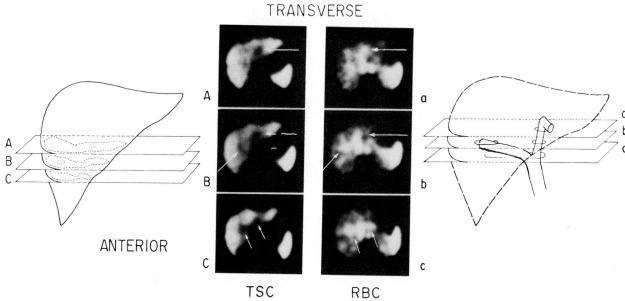

ANTERIOR

TSC   RBC

Case 6–64.—Left and Right Portal Veins Causing Defects on the Transverse Sections of the Emission Computed Tomograms of the Liver

Transverse slices **(A, B** and **C)** of the liver image with Tc-99m sulfur colloid **(TSC)** show defects in the left and right lobe of the liver *(arrows).* Corresponding slices of the blood pool image with Tc-99m red blood cells **(RBC)** show the left and right portal vein **(a & b)** and bifurcation **(c)** that caused the defects on the slices of the **TSC** image.

7

The Hepato-Biliary System

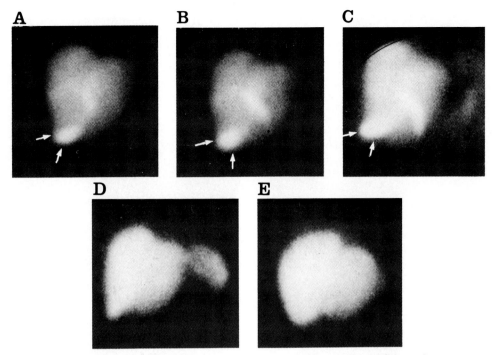

Case 7–1.—Ectopic Gallbladder in the Colic Impression Demonstrated on a Hepatobiliary Scan

Biliary imaging was performed on a 77-year-old woman with abdominal pain using technetium Tc-99m diisopropyl iminodiacetic acid (disofenin).

Sequential images taken at 15 minutes **(A)**, 25 minutes **(B)**, and 35 minutes **(C)** after the injection show the gallbladder at the inferior tip of the right lobe *(arrows)*. A liver scan obtained on the same patient using technetium Tc-99m sulfur colloid, anterior **(D)** and right anterior oblique **(E)** views, showed no evidence of an intrahepatic space-occupying structure in the tip of the right lobe. The findings from the two scans showed that the ectopic gallbladder is not intrahepatic but lies in the colonic impression. An ultrasonogram revealed obstruction of common bile duct and normal gallbladder, a rare form of normal variant in the position of the gallbladder.

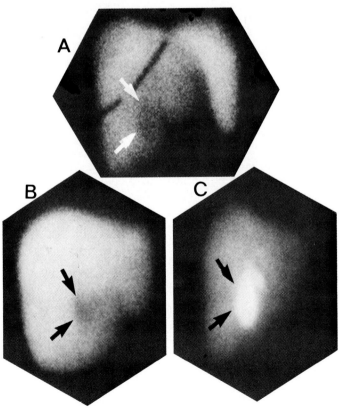

Case 7–2.—Intrahepatic Gallbladder Causing a Defect on a Liver Scan; Example Case 1

Liver-spleen scan obtained using technetium Tc-99m sulfur colloid on a 32-year-old woman with known sickle cell disease and clinically suspected liver abscess.

A, anterior view shows a large defect in the inferior liver, above the usual gallbladder fossa *(white arrows)*.

B, right anterior oblique view shows the defect more convincingly *(black arrows)*.

C, the anterior oblique view taken after an injection of technetium Tc-99m paraisopropyl iminodiacetic acid (iprofenin, or PIPIDA) reveals that the intrahepatic gallbladder caused the "defect" on the liver image *(black arrows)*.

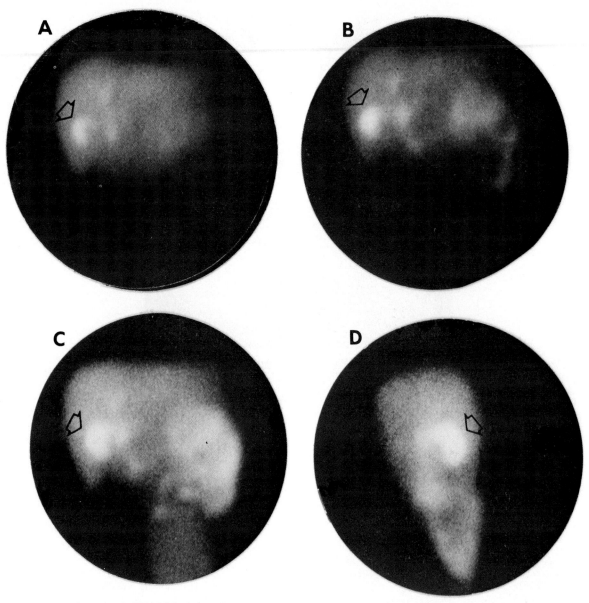

Case 7–3.—Intrahepatic Gallbladder; Example Case 2

The biliary scintigraphy was performed on a 29-year-old man with sickle cell anemia who developed abdominal pain and rising bilirubin level in the plasma.

The sequential images were obtained after an intravenous dose of technetium Tc-99m disofenin. **A,** 15-minute image showing intrahepatic duct and the gallbladder embedded in the right lobe of the liver. **B,** 25-minute image; **C,** 45-minute image; and **D,** right lateral view taken to confirm the intrahepatic gallbladder *(arrows).*

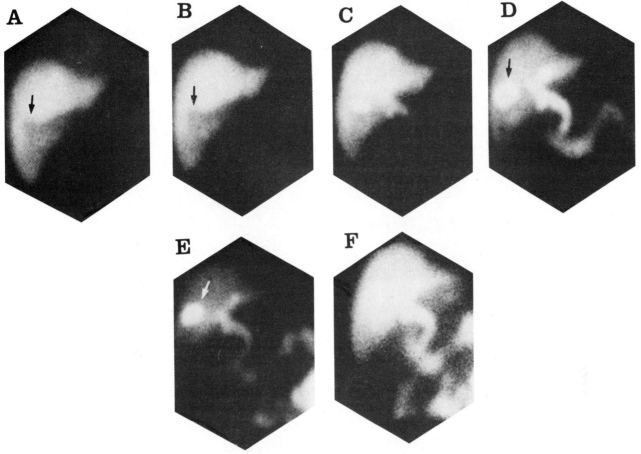

Case 7–4.—Intrahepatic Gallbladder in the Right Lobe That May Cause a Defect in the Liver on an Early Hepatobiliary Scan; Example Case 3

Hepatobiliary scan was obtained using technetium Tc-99m disofenin on a 61-year-old man with history of chronic cholecystitis.

Anterior five-minute **(A)** and ten-minute **(B)** images show normal liver uptake and large "defect" in the inferior right lobe of the liver *(arrows)*. Twenty-minute **(C)** and 40-minute **(D)** images show the gallbladder in the right lobe *(arrows)*, corresponding to the "liver defect" seen on the early images. A 60-minute image shows retention of the radionuclide in the gallbladder **(E)**. There is normal excretion into the intestine immediately after a fatty meal **(F)**; a common finding in patients with a long history of dilated gallbladder or who have fasted longer than 48 hours.

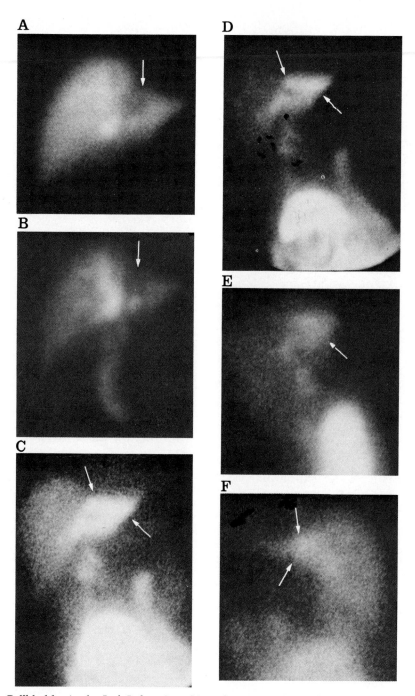

Case 7–5.—Ectopic Gallbladder in the Left Lobe of the Liver Seen on a Hepatobiliary Scan

Hepatobiliary scan was performed on a 55-year-old man with recent history of abdominal colic pain and jaundice, using technetium Tc-99m disofenin. He had a similar episode two years earlier and underwent a cholecystectomy. However, the surgeon could not find the gallbladder. He was referred to us for the biliary study. Ultrasonogram showed dilated biliary ducts but no gallbladder in the gallbladder fossa. Serial biliary images taken at five minutes **(A)** and 25 minutes **(B)** show dilated bile ducts and normal excretion into the intestine.

In addition, a large defect is noted in the superior medial aspect of the left lobe *(arrow)*. Delayed images obtained at two hours **(C)** and 2.5 hours **(D)** show collection of the radioactivity in the superior left lobe region *(arrows)*. Right anterior oblique **(E)** and posterior **(F)** views confirm the collection of radionuclide in the superior left lobe, above the gastric impression that appeared as a defect on the early images **(A** and **B).** The findings indicate chronic cholecystitis of an ectopic gallbladder in the superior left lobe, an extremely rare variant.

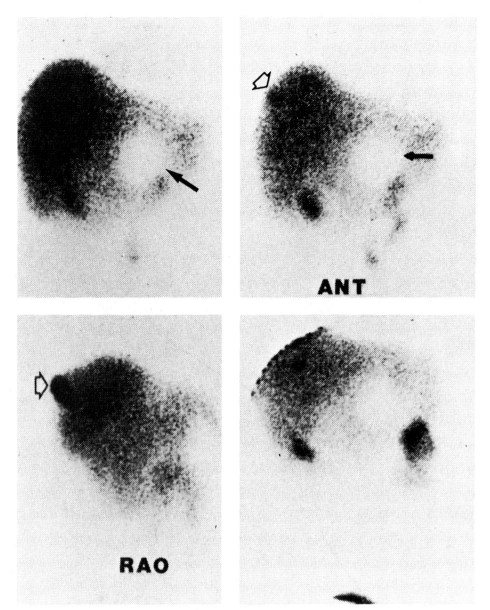

Case 7–6.—Suprahepatic Gallbladder

Cholescintigraphy was performed on a 52-year-old man with suspected cholecystitis using technetium Tc-99m iprofenin (PIPIDA). The images show an area of intense focal uptake in the lateral dome of the liver *(open arrow)*. An ectopic gallbladder without disease was found at operation in the right subdiaphragmatic region corresponding to the scan finding.

A large, round photon-deficient area in the left lobe of the liver *(solid arrow)* represented a 6-cm sterile abscess that was drained at the surgery.

(Courtesy of Youngwirth L.D., Peters, J.C., Perry, M.C., et al. [Guthrie Clinic, Packer Hospital, Sayre, Pennsylvania]: The suprahepatic gall bladder. *Radiology* 149:57, 1983.)

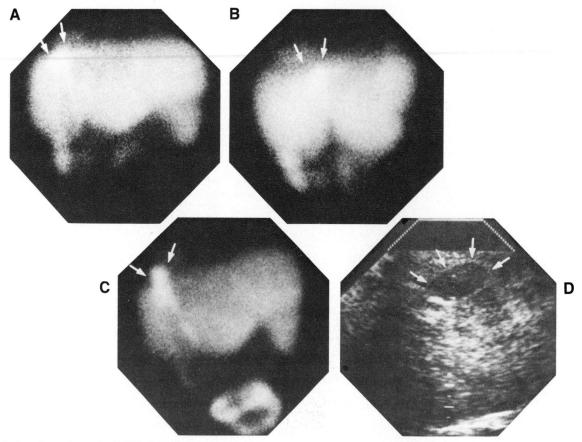

Case 7–7.—Suprahepatic Gallbladder; Example Case 2

Hepatobiliary images were obtained on a 61-year-old woman with breast carcinoma, one hour after the technetium Tc-99m sulfur colloid scan of the liver and spleen, because linear defects noted on the scan in the posterior liver were suspected to be ectopic biliary system. The anterior (**A**) and right anterior oblique (**B**) views taken 20 minutes after and an anterior view taken one hour after (**C**) an intravenous injection of technetium Tc-99m disofenin show an ectopic gallbladder *(white arrows)* and bile ducts.

An ultrasonogram (**D**) confirmed the ectopic gallbladder in the posterior dome of the liver.

(Comment: incidence of ectopic gallbladder or intrahepatic gallbladder is not high. However, such ectopic gallbladder causes defect in the liver scan and may result in a falsely positive scan interpretation, especially in patients with known malignancy.)

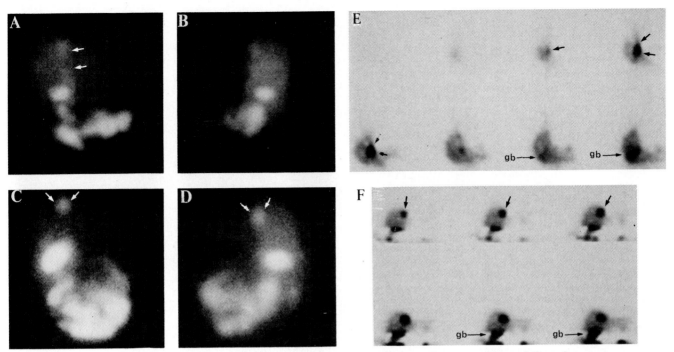

Case 7–8.—Hepatic Adenoma Mimics a "Second Gallbladder" or "Biliary Cyst" on a Hepatobiliary Scan

Hepatobiliary scan was obtained on a 35-year-old woman with clinically suspected acute cholecystitis, using a 5-mCi dose of technetium Tc-99m disofenin.

Anterior **(A)** and posterior **(B)** images taken 40 minutes after the dose show the activity in the gallbladder and excretion into the intestine. In addition, there was linear activity extending to the dome of the liver *(arrows)*. Delayed images, anterior **(C)** and posterior **(D)** views, taken one hour after the dose showed distended gallbladder, with most of the activity being in the intestine. Another focus of radioactivity collection was noted in the dome of the liver *(arrows)*.

The finding was thought to be attributable to a second gallbladder or an anomalous biliary cyst. The focal collection of the radioactivity in the dome of the liver, forming a round mass or sac, was confirmed by the emission computed tomography, transverse sections **(E)** and coronal sections **(F)**, but the "second gallbladder" was found to be a hepatic adenoma *(black arrows)*, which developed after long history of oral estrogen use *(gb:* gallbladder).

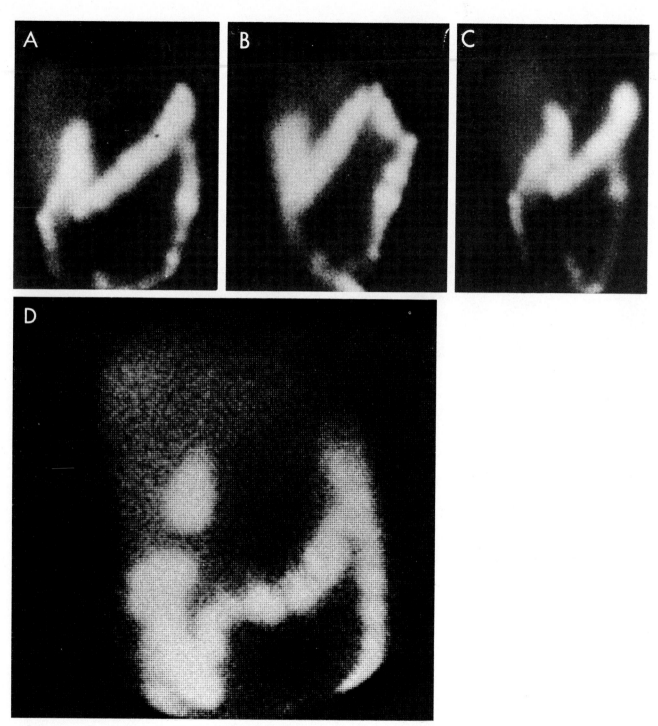

Case 7–9.—Standing up for Cholescintigraphy to Demonstrate Hidden Gallbladder

Hepatobiliary images were obtained on a 23-year-old woman with clinically suspected cholecystitis. The first two-hour sequential images were inconclusive. The delayed images were obtained 17 hours after the injection. Anterior **(A)**, left anterior oblique **(B)**, and right anterior oblique views **(C)** show intestinal activity but failed to separate possible gallbladder activity from the colonic activity.

A repeated imaging with patient standing **(D)** shows clear separation of the gallbladder activity from the colonic activity.

This case illustrates the utility of the upright image in visualizing the gallbladder when it is obscured by overlying colonic activity during cholescintigraphy.

(Courtesy of Growcock G., Lecklitner M.L. [University of Texas Health Science Center, San Antonio, Texas]: Standing up for cholescintigraphy. *Clin. Nucl. Med.* 8:379, 1983.)

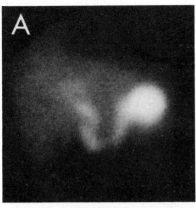 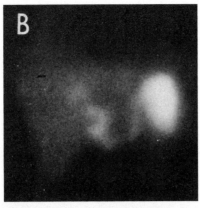 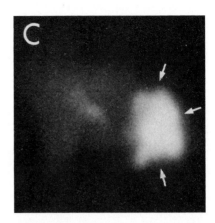

Case 7–10.—Reflux of Hepatobiliary Imaging Agent Into the Stomach

Hepatobiliary scan was obtained using technetium Tc-99m disofenin on a 28-year-old woman with sudden onset of epigastric pain, nausea, and vomiting. Endoscopy revealed gastritis with bile in the stomach.

The scan, anterior image at 45 minutes **(A),** shows excretion of the radionuclide through the bile ducts. The intense activity collection in the left lobe region suggests possible intrahepatic gallbladder in the left lobe.

Another anterior image taken at one hour **(B)** shows continued drainage of the radioactivity into the left upper quadrant "sac."

Gallbladder was not visualized throughout the study.

Immediately after the one-hour image, the patient was given a glass (6 oz.) of carbonated soft drink (7-Up), and the same view image was taken **(C).** The repeated image after the 7-Up shows enlarged *(arrows)* volume of the "sac" indicating it is the stomach.

(Comment: localization, normal or abnormal, of a radionuclide in the stomach can be confirmed by such "Coke test" or "7-Up test" easily.)

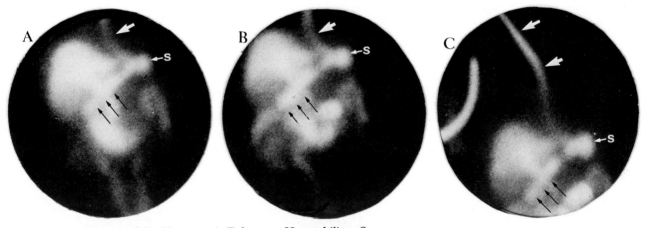

Case 7–11.—Images of the Nasogastric Tube on a Hepatobiliary Scan

Hepatobiliary scan was obtained using technetium Tc-99m disofenin on a 84-year-old woman with sudden onset of nausea, vomiting, and abdominal pain. Twenty- **(A)** and 30-minute **(B)** scans show normal uptake by the liver and normal excretion into the intestine. However, there was linear activity below the liver that extended upward through the left upper quadrant and into the thorax. Anterior image over the chest **(C)** was taken to trace the linear activity and disclosed that the upward activity extension was the radionuclide reflux through the nasogastric tube, the tip of which was in the duodenum *(black arrows)*. The tube was twisted in the stomach *(s)* and ran through the esophagus *(white arrows)*. The external part of the tube is also filled partly with the radioactive agent **(C).**

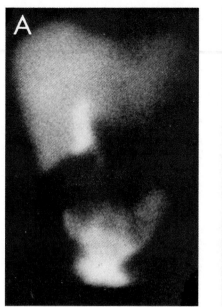 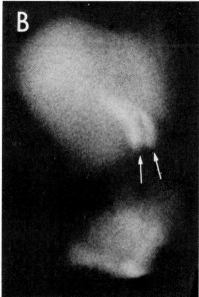 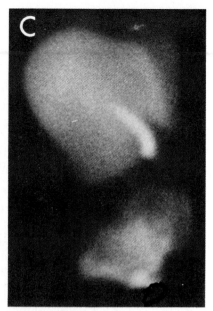

Case 7–12.—Double Common Bile Duct on a Hepatobiliary Scan Caused by a Yawn; A Motion Artifact

Anterior hepatobiliary image obtained two hours after an intravenous injection of technetium Tc-99m disofenin on a 16-year-old boy with hyperbilirubinemia **(A)** shows normal liver uptake, delayed excretion into the intestine, and high activity retention in the common bile duct.

A right anterior oblique view **(B)** shows a double common bile duct *(arrows)*.

A repeated oblique view taken immediately after the **B** image shows only one common bile duct. The patient yawned during the first oblique view imaging. Movement of the liver during yawning is responsible for the double image of the common bile duct and the less clear outline of the liver.

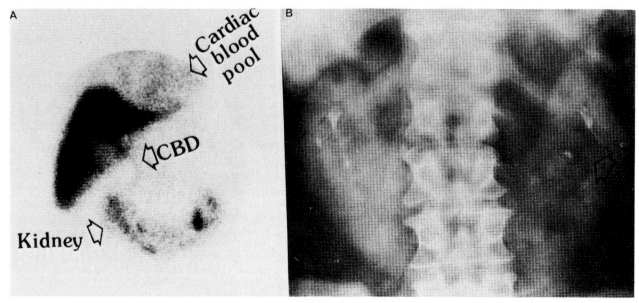

Case 7–13.—Horseshoe Kidney Simulating Excretion of Radionuclide Into the Intestine on a Biliary Scan

A hepatobiliary scan was obtained on a 67-year-old man with jaundice and abnormal liver function test results. An anterior image **(A)** taken ten minutes after an injection of technetium Tc-99m iprofenin shows persistent cardiac blood pool activity, visualization of the common bile duct, and a horseshoe kidney, which mimics intestinal activity. An intravenous pyelogram **(B)** confirms the presence of horseshoe kidney *(arrow)*.

(Courtesy of Delong S.R. [Forbes Health System, Monroeville, Pennsylvania]: Incidental findings on a single Tc-99m PIPIDA scan. *Clin. Nucl. Med.* 8:90, 1983.)

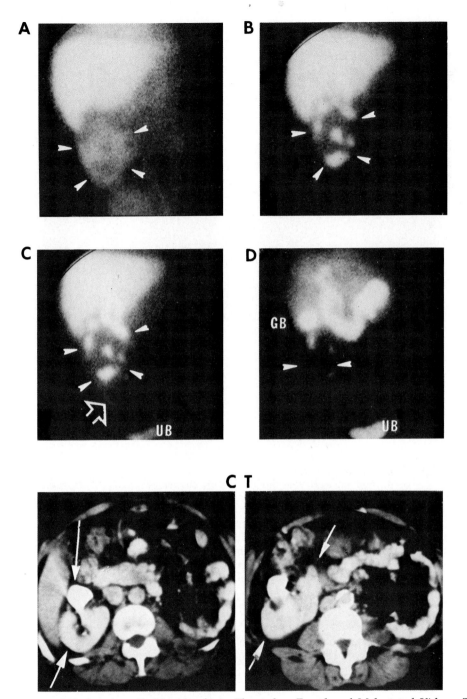

Case 7–14.—Excretion of Technetium Tc-99m disofenin Through a Fused and Malrotated Kidney That Mimics the Excretion of the Biliary Agent Into the Intestine

A, hepatobiliary scan obtained on a 43-year-old woman with acute abdominal pain, one-minute image, shows a large, round "mass" which concentrates the radiopharmaceutical *(arrowheads).*

B, 15-minute image showing excretion of the radiopharmaceutical; appearance of intestinal activity *(arrowheads).*

C, 30-minute image shows a drainage of the radioactive agent into the urinary bladder *(open arrow and UB).*

D, almost complete clearance of the activity from the "mass" and increased concentration of the radioactive agent in the urinary bladder *(UB)*. The gallbladder *(GB)* and true excretion of the radiopharmaceutical into the intestine was visualized.

CT, computed tomography of the abdomen showing a fused and malrotated kidney in the right lower quadrant corresponding to the "mass" seen on the biliary images.

(Comment: when accumulation of the radioactivity is noted in the urinary bladder on a hepatobiliary scan, probable visualization of the renal calices and/or ureter should be anticipated, and excretion of the radiopharmaceutical through the renal system should be carefully differentiated from the excretion into the intestine.)

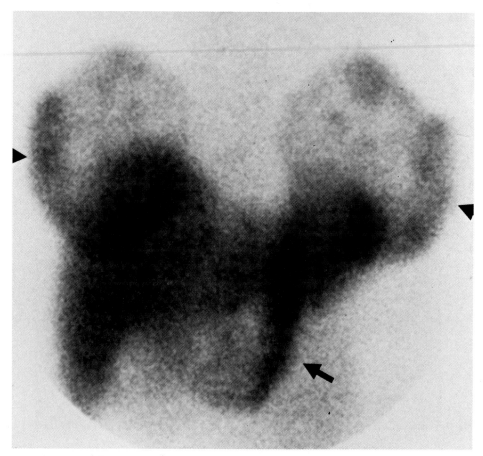

Case 7–15.—Breast Uptake of Tc-99m iprofenin

Hepatobiliary scan was performed on a 21-year-old man with suspected biliary obstruction, using 7-mCi dose of technetium Tc-99m iprofenin. The abdominal image taken three hours after the injection shows unexpected and persistent localization of the radionuclide in both breasts *(arrows)*. There is linear uptake in the left upper abdomen, which represents a displaced bowel secondary to laparotomy performed for an abdominal stab wound *(arrow)*.

The cause of such intense breast uptake was not documented; however, medical history and physical examination revealed that the patient is a transvestite and has been taking a large but undisclosed amount of conjugated estrogens. He had a marked breast tissue development bilaterally without surgical implants or inflammations.

(Courtesy of Moreno A.J., Coffey W.A., Brown J.M., et al. [William Beaumont Army Medical Center, El Paso, Texas]: Unexpected breast uptake of Tc-99m-PIPIDA. *J. Nucl. Med.* 24:861, 1983.)

8

The Kidneys and Abdomen

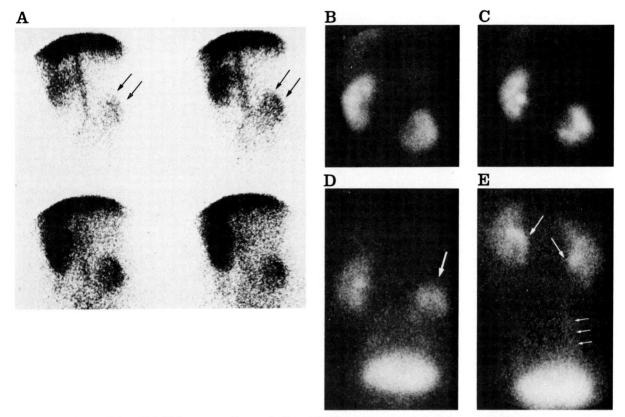

Case 8–1.—Ptotic (Movable) Kidney on a Dynamic Renal Study

Dynamic renal study was performed on a 18-year-old girl with a three-year history of idiopathic hypertension using an intravenous bolus injection of technetium Tc-99m pentetic acid at upright position (sitting). The flow images **(A)** show abnormally decreased right renal arterial flow *(arrows)*. Static images taken at three minutes **(B)** and five minutes **(C)** show relatively even distribution of the radionuclide in both kidneys. A thirty-minute static image **(D)** shows active filtration and excretion of the radioactive agent into the bladder, but the filtration function of the right appears to be impaired *(arrow)*.

Immediately after the 30-minute image, the image was repeated at supine position **(E).** The repeated image at supine position shows a definite improvement of the renal filtration bilaterally with facilitated excretion of the radionuclide from the both kidneys *(arrows)*. An intravenous pyelogram performed on this patient showed normal kidneys bilaterally with a small left caliceal tic.

(Comments: such ptotic kidney is reported to be a frequent cause of orthostatic hypertension [Clorius J.H., Kjelle-Schweigler M., Ostertag H., et al.: [131]Hippuran renography in the detection of orthostatic hypertension. *J. Nucl. Med.* 19:343, 1978]. When one kidney is ptotic with decreased arterial flow, a simple supine image obtained at different positions may reveal invaluable information for the management of the patient.)

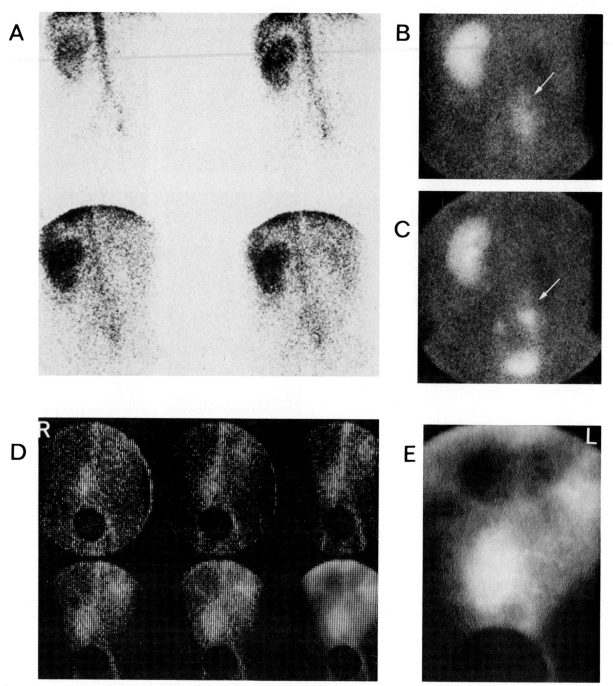

Case 8–2.—Pelvic Kidney; Example Case 1

A 27-year-old man with "malignant hypertension" was known to have "only one kidney." The dynamic renal study with technetium Tc-99m pentetic acid was requested for an evaluation of a recent rise of plasma creatinine level.

A, posterior flow images showed slightly delayed but fairly normal arterial flow to the right kidney. The left kidney was not imaged.

B and **C,** static images at five and 20 minutes showed normal initial uptake and later filtration of the radiopharmaceutical in the right kidney. There was an ectopic focus of radiopharmaceutical collection in the midline pelvis *(thin arrow)*.

D and **E,** anterior flow images of the pelvis and a static image at five minutes showed the "absent right kidney" to be a "pelvic kidney."

(Comments: when a kidney is not visualized on a radionuclide renal study in patient with no history of unilateral renal disease or nephrectomy, a repeated anterior renal flow study becomes the procedure of choice to document ectopic pelvic kidney.)

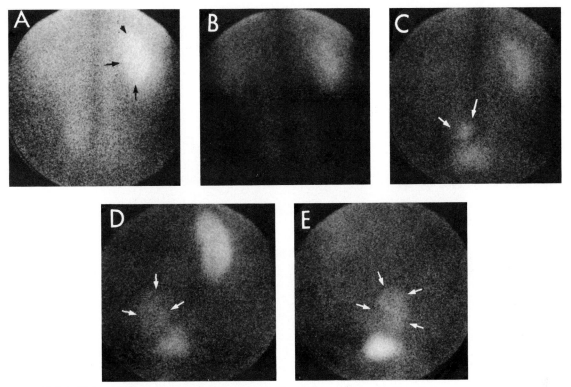

Case 8–3.—Pelvic Kidney Demonstrated on a Dynamic Renal Scan; Example Case 2

Dynamic renal study was performed using technetium Tc-99m pentetic acid on a 35-year-old man who is known to have only one kidney. A posterior image taken one minute after the injection **(A)** shows a normal blood pool activity in the right kidney *(arrows)*. The left kidney is not clearly visualized on the one-minute **(A)** or ten-minute **(B)** views. 30-minute **(C)** and one-hour **(D)** images show clear configuration of the right kidney and nonvisualization of the left kidney. There is collection of radioactivity in the pelvis in a shape that is not attributable to the bladder *(arrows)*. An anterior view of the pelvis shows **(E)** the right kidney lying superior and posterior to the bladder *(arrows)*, a pelvic kidney.

Incidence of such ectopic kidney is known to be one in 2,000 cases (Warkany J.: *Congenital Malformations*. Chicago, Year Book Medical Publishers, 1971, p. 1053).

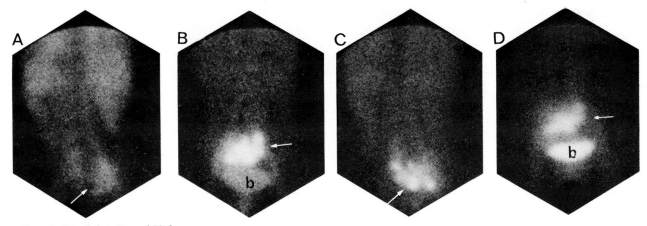

Case 8–4.—Pelvic Fused Kidney

Dynamic renal study was performed on a 24-year-old woman with proteinuria, using intravenous dose of technetium Tc-99m pentetic acid. A posterior image at one minute **(A)** shows no clear images of the kidneys, but there was unusual blood pool activity in the pelvis *(arrow)*.

Anterior image taken at ten minutes **(B)** shows enlarged kidney *(arrow)* above the bladder *(b)*.

A repeated posterior image at one hour **(C)** and an anterior image **(D)** again demonstrate the large, single pelvic kidney—pelvic fused kidney.

Case 8–5.—Intrathoracic Kidney Found on a Radionuclide Renography

Left lateral **(A)** and posterior **(B)** static images taken after an intravenous injection of technetium Tc-99m pentetic acid in a 7-month-old black female. A chest roentgenogram taken earlier showed a soft tissue mass in the right lower chest, and a renal ultrasonography failed to show the right kidney.

The radionuclide image of the kidney showed the right kidney to be located abnormally high, near the heart. *H:* heart, *R:* right kidney, *S:* stomach, LLAT: left lateral, L: left side.

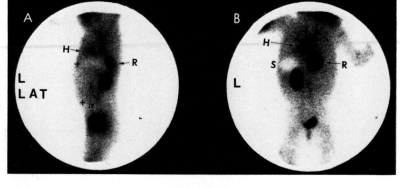

(Courtesy of Williams A. [University of New Mexico, Albuquerque]: Intrathoracic kidney on radionuclide renography. *Clin. Nucl. Med.* 8:409, 1983.)

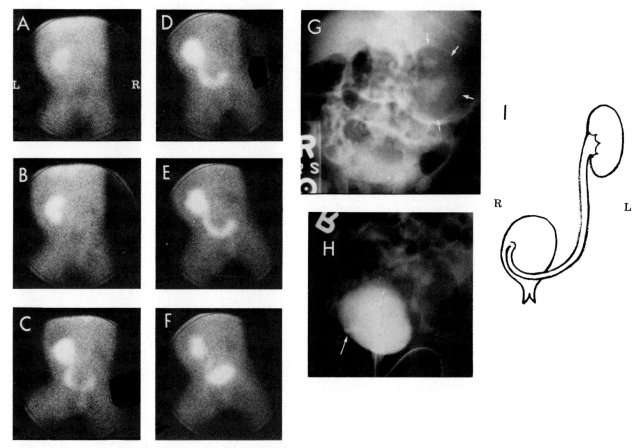

Case 8–6.—Crossed Renal Ectopy With Solitary Kidney Demonstrated on a Dynamic Renal Study

Dynamic renal study was obtained using technetium Tc-99m pentetic acid on a 2-month-old infant girl with cardiac ventricular septal defect and slightly elevated plasma BUN and creatinine levels.

Posterior views taken at 1 minute **(A)**, 5 minutes **(B)**, 15 minutes **(C)**, 25 minutes **(D)**, 35 minutes **(E)**, and 50 minutes **(F)** after the injection show only the left kidney with slightly decreased concentration of the radionuclide. The ureter appears to be dilated, with retention of radioactivity, and the ureter crosses over to the right side of the bladder **(C to E)**. The right kidney was not visualized throughout the study.

An intravenous pyelogram (IVP) **(G)** on the same patient shows slightly hydronephrotic left kidney *(arrows)*. The IVP failed to delineate the right kidney.

A retrograde urogram **(H)** shows a normal bladder and the right ureterovesicular junction *(arrow)*.

Agenesis of the right kidney was later confirmed by an abdominal angiography.

This is an extremely rare case of "crossed renal ectopy with solitary left kidney" (Purpon I.: Crossed renal ectopy with solitary kidney: A review of the literature. *Urology* 90:13, 1963). The anatomy of the anomaly of this case is illustrated **(I)**.

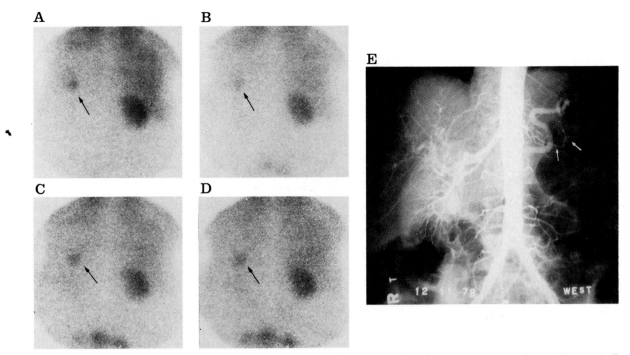

Case 8–7.—Superior Polar Artery Supplying the Upper Pole of the Left Kidney Demonstrated on a Dynamic Renal Study

Dynamic renal study was performed using technetium Tc-99m pentetic acid on a 76-year-old woman with sudden onset of severe left flank pain.

Images at three minutes **(A)**, 7 minutes **(B)**, 20 minutes **(C)**, and 30 minutes **(D)** show fairly normal initial uptake by and filtration through the right kidney and only small functioning focus noted in the left kidney *(arrows)*.

The abdominal aortic angiogram **(E)** shows complete obstruction of the left renal artery. There is a small artery branched off from the aorta and supplies the upper pole of the left kidney, a superior polar artery arising from the aorta.

In the 80% of cases, the superior polar artery arises from the main trunk of the renal artery (Luzsa G.: *X-ray Anatomy of the Vascular System.* Philadelphia, J.B. Lippincott Co., 1974, p. 228).

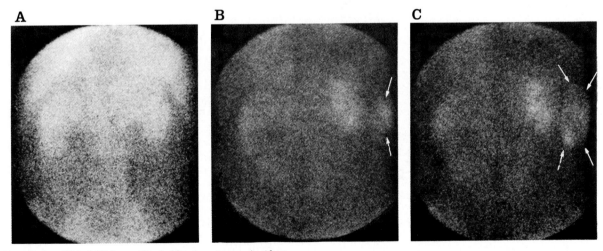

Case 8–8.—Third Kidney (?); A Nephrostomy Artifact

Dynamic renal study was performed using an intravenous dose of technetium Tc-99m pentetic acid on a 64-year-old woman with history of chronic renal failure. A five-minute static image **(A)** shows poor concentration of radionuclide in the kidneys. Fifteen-minute image **(B)** shows an extrarenal collection of radioactivity in the right flank *(arrows)*. Thirty-five-minute image **(C)** shows a third kidney (?) in the right flank, lateral to the right kidney *(arrows)*.

The patient had right nephrostomy, and the third image, mimicking an extra kidney, represented collection of the radioactive urine in the adhesive absorbent dressing over the nephrostomy site.

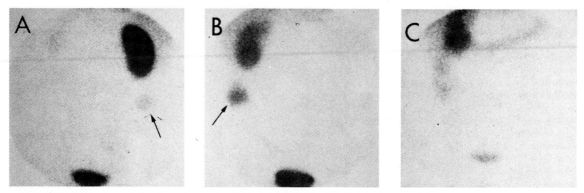

Case 8–9.—Visualization of the Intestine on a Renal Scan; A Radiopharmaceutical Artifact

Posterior renal scan obtained using technetium Tc-99m gluceptate (gluco-heptonate) on a 59-year-old man four hours after the injection **(A)** shows normal uptake by the right kidney. There is minimum activity in the left kidney. In addition, a small area of questionable radioactivity collection is seen below the inferior pole of the right kidney **(A, arrow)**.

An anterior image taken immediately following the posterior view shows that the extrarenal collection of the radioactivity is anteriorly located **(B, arrow)**. A delayed anterior image taken nine hours after the injection **(C)** reveals that the extrarenal activity represents radioactivity excretion into the intestine.

When a renal scan is obtained with technetium Tc-99m gluceptate, such intestinal activity on a delayed image may cause a false impression of a urinoma.

(Courtesy of William B. Martin, M.D., Division of Nuclear Medicine, Department of Radiology, University of Chicago, Chicago.)

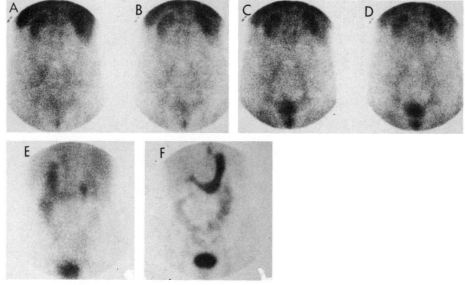

Case 8–10.—Localization of Radionuclide in the Gastrointestinal Tracts Demonstrated on a Renal Scan; Radiopharmaceutical Artifact Due to Poor Quality Control

Dynamic renal study was performed using technetium Tc-99m gluceptate on a 49-year-old woman with chronic renal failure.

Posterior images taken at one **(A)** and three minutes **(B),** and 20 **(C)** and 25 minutes **(D)** show decreased renal concentration and excretion with increased background activity. A delayed posterior image taken at two hours **(E)** shows abnormally decreased renal cortical activity and intense extrarenal activity. A delayed anterior image taken immediately after the delayed posterior image shows intense radioactivity in the stomach and intestine.

Such extrarenal localization of radioactivity in the gastrointestinal tract indicate a poor radiopharmaceutical quality control; high fraction of unbound technetium Tc-99m activity.

Such artifacts due to poor-quality radiopharmaceutical make a proper evaluation of the study difficult and may cause false scan interpretations.

(Contribution by William B. Martin, M.D., Division of Nuclear Medicine, Department of Radiology, University of Chicago Hospital, Chicago.)

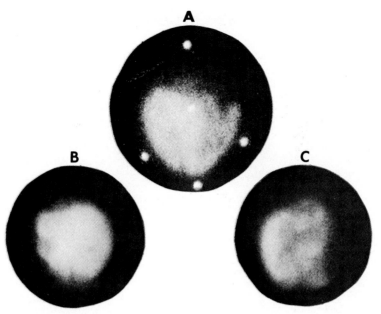

Case 8–11.—Radionuclide Peritoneography; Example Case 1:

Radionuclide peritoneography is performed in order to evaluate patency of the peritoneal cavity. In patient with diffuse malignant process in the abdomen, intraperitoneal injection of chemotherapeutic agents or chromic phosphate P 32 colloid is a recommended procedure. When there is severe adhesion of the peritoneum, the chemotherapeutic agents or the radioactive colloid might be localized in a nontargeted region.

Case 1: Radionuclide peritoneography was performed in a young women who had bilateral breast carcinoma and recently was found to have malignant ascites. The anterior and right and left lateral views of the abdomen were obtained with a large-field-of-view camera after intraperitoneal injection of 5% dextrose in water, 300 ml, followed by a 1-mCi dose of technetium Tc-99m sulfur colloid. Hot markers were placed over the xyphoid, umbilicus, bilateral iliac crests, and over the pubis for the anterior view image. The scans show diffuse, relatively uniform distribution of the radionuclide, indicating a satisfactory patency of the peritoneal cavity. (**A,** anterior; **B,** right lateral; **C,** left lateral views.)

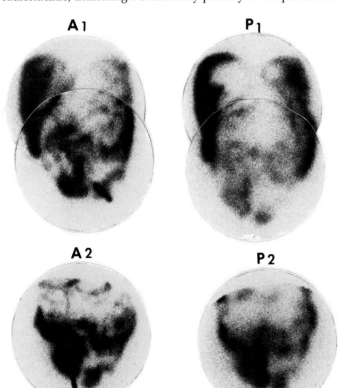

Case 8–12.—Normal Radionuclide Peritoneography; Example Case 2:

Radionuclide peritoneography was performed after an infusion of 500 ml of dextrose in saline through an intraperitoneal catheter followed by an injection of a 1–2-mCi dose of technetium Tc-99m sulfur colloid. The patient had ovarian carcinoma that was surgically excised. During the surgery, it was confirmed that peritoneal cavity was patent without adhesions.

The initial images, anterior (**A₁**) and posterior (**P₁**) views, were taken while the patient was at supine position. Images taken at upright position (**A₂** and **P₂**) show that the radionuclide in dextrose/saline moves freely in the peritoneal cavity ensuring patency of the cavity (compare with Example Case 3).

(Courtesy of Hussein M. Abdel-Dayem, M.D., Professor, Department of Radiology and Nuclear Medicine, Faculty of Medicine, Kuwait University, Safat, Kuwait.)

P-32-COLLOID

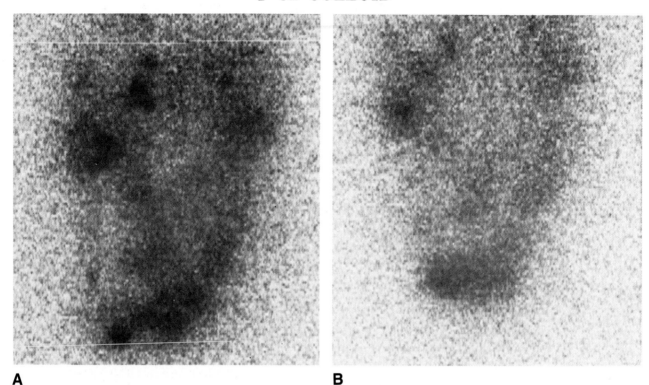

A **B**

Case 8–13.—Bremsstrahlung Peritoneography; An Abnormal Radionuclide Peritoneography

Anterior view peritoneal scan obtained 12 hours **(A)** and 72 hours **(B)** after an intraperitoneal injection of a 10-mCi dose of chromic phosphate P 32 colloid in a patient with disseminated ovarian carcinoma. The scans were taken using a rectilinear scanner with wide window, 50 keV–560 keV, accumulating the bremsstrahlung radiation. The scans show that the distribution of the radionuclide has essentially been unchanged during the 60 hours of the ambulatory period.

The findings indicate diffuse adhesions of radiocolloid in the peritoneum.

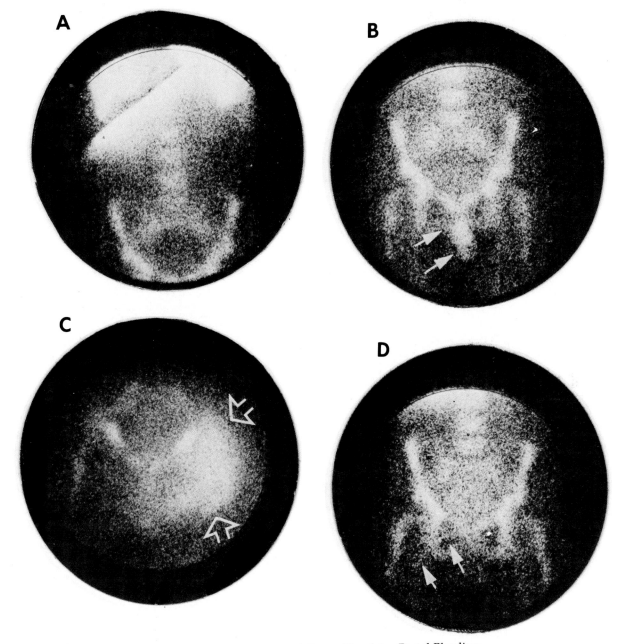

Case 8–14.—Localization of Radiocolloid in the Genital Organ Simulates Rectal Bleeding

Gastrointestinal bleeding study was performed on a 43-year-old man who had an episode of rectal bleeding two days earlier.

A, wrong positioning of the patient. Anterior view of abdomen taken after a slow infusion of a 6-mCi dose of technetium Tc-99m sulfur colloid. The liver is shielded. When the bleeding is suspected to be from the rectum, the imaging view should include the region below the pubis.

B, anterior view pelvis, correct positioning for the detection of rectal bleeding. An area of abnormal localization is noted midline, below the pubis (arrows). The finding may suggest rectal bleeding. However, the localization could also be in the genital organ.

Additional views to localize the abnormal uptake:

C, SOC (sit-on-camera) view. This view can clearly differentiate an anterior pelvic lesion from a posterior lesion. Diffuse activity seen on the right (open arrows) is the activity from the liver.

D, when the uptake is suspected to be in the genital organ, a repeated image may be obtained while the penis is taped aside (arrows).

9

The Vascular System

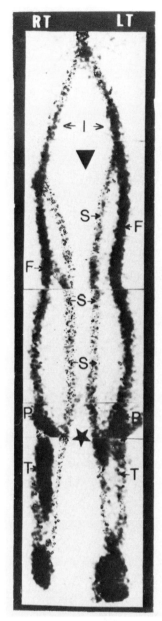

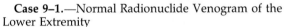

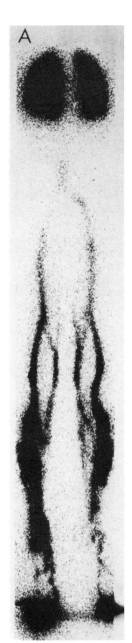

Case 9–1.—Normal Radionuclide Venogram of the Lower Extremity

Lower extremity radionuclide venogram obtained using technetium Tc-99m macroaggregated albumin, 2 mCi in an average volume of 0.2 ml, injected into the bilateral dorsal metatarsal veins.

The composite image from images over the calves, the lower thigh, the upper thigh, over the lower pelvis and over the upper pelvis, shows the iliac veins (*I*), the femoral veins (*F*), the great saphenous system (*S*), the popliteal veins (*P*), and the tibial veins (*T*).

Case 9–2.—Normal Lower Body Venography Performed Using a Whole Body Imaging System

Lower body venography was performed using a moving table and a large-field-of-view gamma camera, and with technetium Tc-99m macroaggregated albumin. The dose was injected into the bilateral dorsal metatarsal veins, and the flow of the radionuclide through the deep and superficial veins to the lungs was imaged by the whole body imaging system **(A).**

The venogram shows the posterior perfusion lung image, inferior vena cava, iliac veins, femoral veins, saphenous veins, popliteal veins, and calf veins. Resolution of the calf veins is less than optimum on this venogram with a whole body imaging system.

The second run, delayed image **(B),** shows areas of retention of the radionuclide.

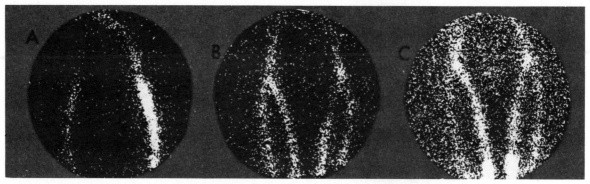

Case 9–3.—Effect of Tourniquet Pressure and the Injection on the Radionuclide Venogram

When there is difference in the tourniquet pressure applied to each leg, the radionuclide flow may be seen earlier, with higher radioactivity from the leg with lighter pressure than the flow from the contralateral side. The visualization of the veins can be markedly delayed when the pressure is tighter than optimum **(A)**.

Proper tourniquet pressure and release of the tourniquet at the proper time allows optimum visualization of the deep veins as well as the saphenous veins **(B)**.

When the below-knee tourniquet is not tight enough, the radionuclide flow becomes mainly through the superficial veins. Thus, flow through the femoral veins may appear as diminished or blocked **(C)**.

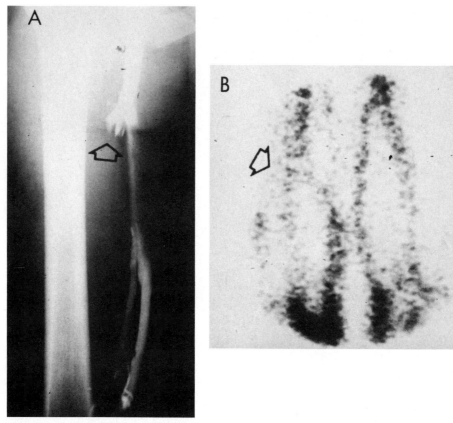

Case 9–4.—Triple Femoral Vein Demonstrated on a Lower Extremity Radionuclide Venogram

Radionuclide venogram over the thigh using technetium Tc-99m macroaggregated albumin **(B)** shows multiple venous flow channels in the right thigh *(open arrow)*, suggesting probable collateral channels, while normal femoral and saphenous veins are visualized in the left thigh.

A contrast venography over the right thigh shows **(A)** a triple femoral vein *(open arrow)*, a frequently seen variant. Two femoral veins (21%) or multiple femoral veins (14%) are known as relatively common variants (Luzsa G.: *X-ray Anatomy of the Vascular System.* Philadelphia, J.B. Lippincott Co., 1974, p. 306). Such a variant may cause a false interpretation as abnormal collateral flows on a radionuclide venogram.

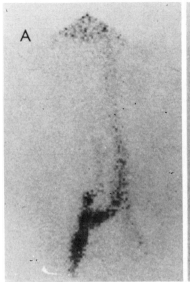
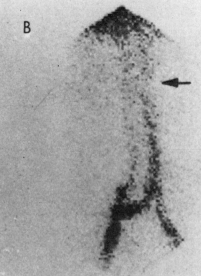

Case 9–5.—Double Inferior Vena Cava
Venogram of the abdominal region
obtained after the injection of sodium
pertechnetate Tc-99m into veins of both
feet on a 57-year-old man with suspected
renal failure. Left and right venae cavae
are seen, which anastomose at the renal
level (arrow).
A, 40–50 seconds; B, 50–60 seconds.
(Courtesy of Rivera J.V., Ficek M.A.
[V.A. Medical and Regional Office, San
Juan, Puerto Rico]: Double inferior vena
cava and anomalous venous drainage from
the left arm demonstration by radionuclide
angiogram. Clin. Nucl. Med. 8:306, 1983.)

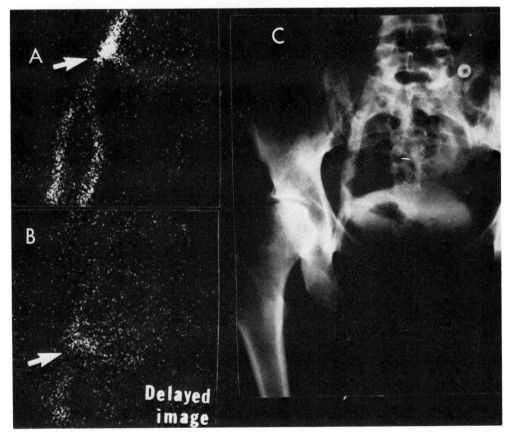

Case 9–6.—Nonspecific Retention of Radionuclide in a Major Deep Vein Seen on a Radionuclide Venogram of the
Pelvis
Radionuclide venogram of the pelvis was obtained using technetium Tc-99m macroaggregated albumin injected into
a dorsal metatarsal vein.
A static image over the pelvis at later phase, ten minutes after the injection, shows an intense radioactivity retention
in the iliac vein (A, arrow). A delayed view obtained an hour later shows a mild but persistent retention of the radionuclide in the iliac vein (B, arrow). A contrast venography of the right iliac vein (C) shows normal iliac vein. However,
suggestive findings of partial compression of the vein were noted at the junction of the common iliac vein and inferior
vena cava (arrow).

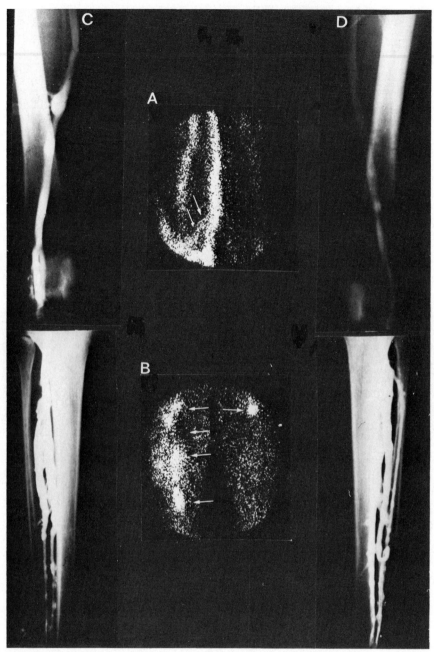

Case 9–7.—Popliteal and Saphenous Vein Anastomosis and Nonspecific "Hot Spots" on a Radionuclide Venogram
    Radionuclide venogram over the bilateral popliteal region **(A)** shows an unusual venous channel connecting the popliteal and the saphenous vein in the left lower leg *(arrows)*. Such unusual communications or branchings are very common variants in the lower extremity veins. A delayed static view over the calf shows multiple "hot spots" in the right calf and a single "hot spot" in the left calf **(B,** *arrows)*.
    Contrast venography performed on the right **(C)** and left leg **(D)** showed essentially normal venous system.

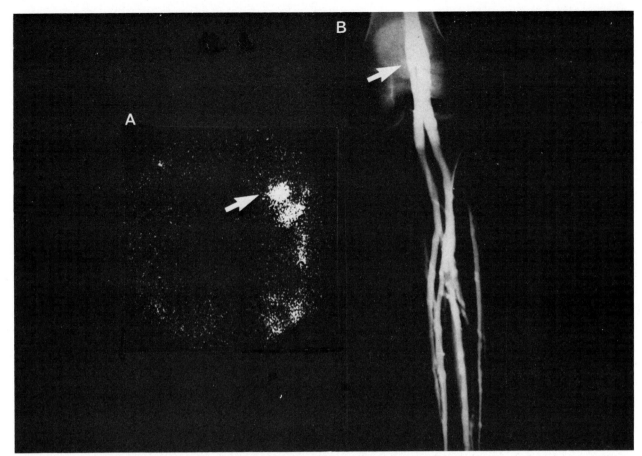

Case 9–8.—Retention or Adherence of Technetium Tc-99m Macroaggregated Albumin Around the Venous Valves
Delayed, static image of radionuclide venogram of the left leg obtained using technetium Tc-99m macroaggregated albumin shows multiple "hot spots" in the calf **(A).** The contrast venogram of the leg **(B)** shows that the most intense hot spot corresponds to the region of popliteal venous valve *(arrow)*. The findings suggest that the valve is tagged by the technetium Tc-99m macroaggregated albumin. However, an in vivo experiment failed to demonstrate adherence of the particles to the venous valves (Ryo U.Y., Colonbetti L.G., Polin S.G., et al.: Radionuclide venography: Significance of delayed washout; visualization of the saphenous system. *J. Nucl. Med.* 17:590, 1976).

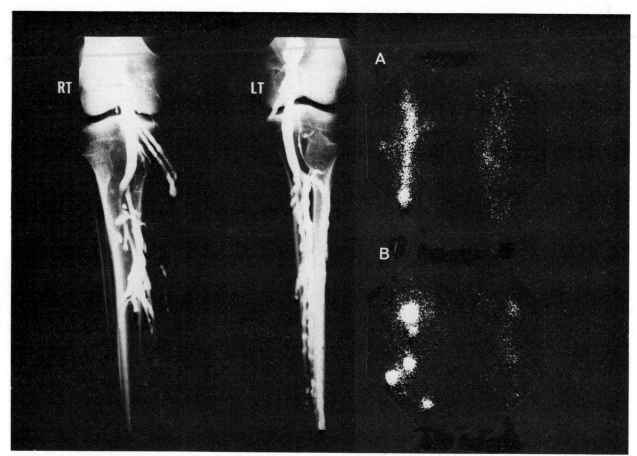

Case 9–9.—Aggregation of Technetium Tc-99m Macroaggregated Albumin in a Normal Vein Causing "Hot Spots" on Radionuclide Venogram

Radionuclide venogram, static image over the calves, taken at later phase (ten minutes after injection) shows normal clearance from the left calf and abnormal retention in the right calf region **(A).** A delayed image that was taken one hour later shows multiple "hot spots" **(B).** These hot spots were not seen on an earlier image.

The findings suggest aggregation of the radioactive particles in a vein, which probably has venous stasis and turbulence.

Contrast venogram over both calves shows normal venous system of the calves *(left).*

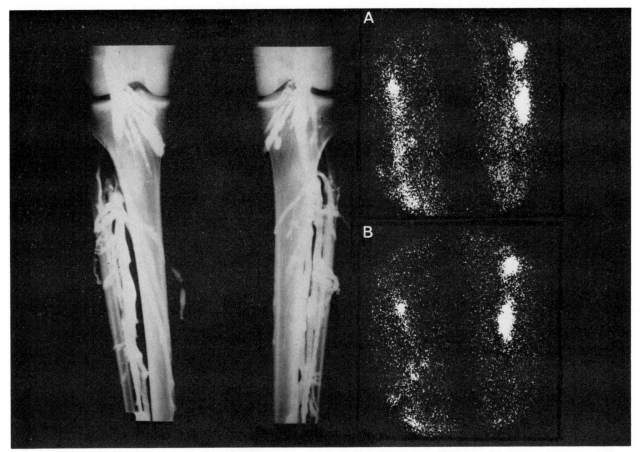

Case 9–10.—Persistent "Hot Spots" on a Radionuclide Venogram of Normal Calf Veins

Later phase, static radionuclide venogram obtained over the calves ten minutes after injections of technetium Tc-99m macroaggregated albumin **(A)** shows multiple "hot spots" in the both calves. A delayed image obtained one hour later shows almost same "hot spots" in the same location as on the earlier image. These hot spots remained at the same location, though patient walked around for a while.

Contrast venogram of the both calves, however, shows normal venous system *(left)*.

"Hot spots" alone in the calf region, therefore, do not represent thrombosis or other venous abnormality but are essentially a nonspecific finding (Ryo U.Y., Quazi M., Srikantaswamy S., et al.: Radionuclide venography: Correlation with contrast venography. *J. Nucl. Med.* 18:11, 1977).

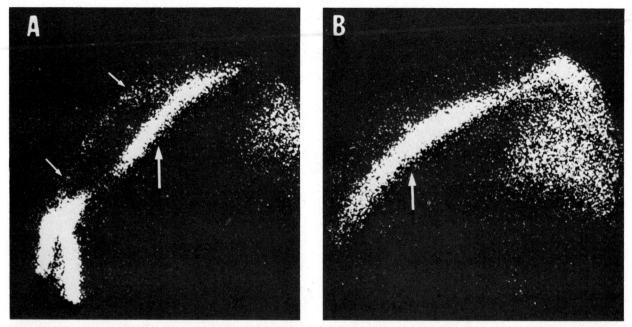

Case 9–11.—Normal Upper Extremity Venogram; Example Case 1

Radionuclide venogram of the arm obtained using technetium Tc-99m macroaggregated albumin shows the cephalic vein *(thin arrows),* and brachial vein *(thick arrow)* on an early image **(A).** Normal deep veins and brachial vein draining into the axillary vein are imaged on a later phase image **(B).** Trapping of the technetium Tc-99m macroaggregated albumin in the lung is also imaged.

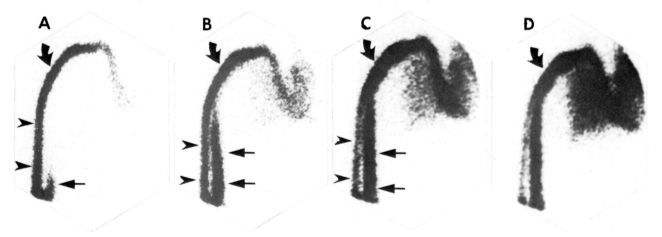

Case 9–12.—Normal Upper Extremity Venogram; Example Case 2

Upper extremity venogram, an early flow image taken immediately after an injection of technetium Tc-99m macroaggregated albumin through the distal cephalic vein and a release of tourniquet shows **(A)** normal flow through the cephalic vein *(arrowheads)* and axillary vein *(curved arrow).*

Images obtained at later phase show gradually increasing radioactivity flow through the brachial vein *(straight arrows).* A gradual accumulation of the radionuclide in the lung is visualized on the later image.

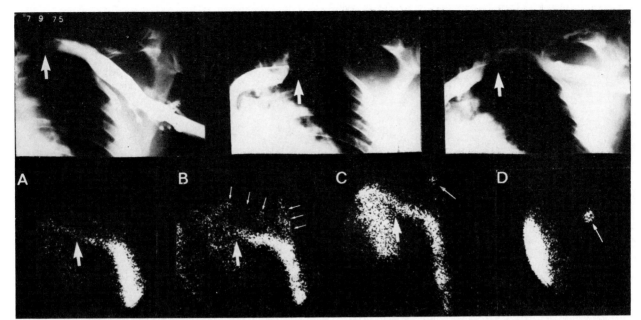

Case 9–13.—Hypertrophic Valve Causing Sign of Deep Vein Obstruction on an Upper Extremity Venogram

Radionuclide venography performed using technetium Tc-99m macroaggregated albumin on a left arm with history of intermittent edema shows flow obstruction in the axillary vein (**A** and **B**, *thick arrow*) and collateral channels (**B**, *thin arrows*). When the arm was stretched and rotated externally, the axillary vein became open (**C**, *thick arrow*).

A delayed image showed a trapping of radioparticles in the region of the deltoid muscle, indicating trapping of the particles at the capillary level of the collateral channels.

A contrast venography of the left arm **(top)**, anterior and oblique views, shows a hypertrophic valve of the axillary vein that caused functional obstruction of the axillary vein with formations of collateral channels.

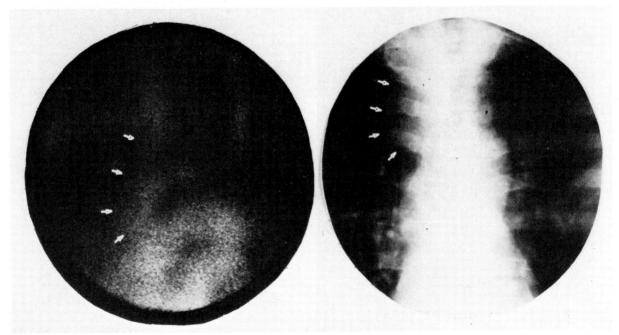

Case 9–14.—Anomalous Origin of the Innominate Artery Causing a "Mass" in the Superior Mediastinum Detected on a Radionuclide Angiogram

A radionuclide angiogram over the upper mediastinum was obtained on a 75-year-old man with a possible "mass" in the superior mediastinum (**right,** *arrows*), using technetium Tc-99m red blood cells labeled by means of in vitro labeling technique.

A pinhole image of the angiogram shows an abnormal origin of the innominate artery, originated from the ascending aorta, that corresponds to the superior mediastinum "mass" (**left,** *arrows*).

Such anomalous origin of the innominate artery is a relatively common variant (Warkany J.: *Congenital Malformations.* Chicago, Year Book Medical Publishers, 1971, p. 529).

THE VASCULAR SYSTEM **153**

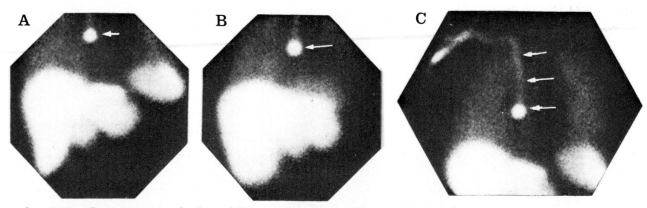

Case 9–15.—Demonstration of a Central Venous Catheter on a Liver and Spleen Scan

Anterior view **(A)** and right anterior oblique view **(B)** liver and spleen scan obtained using technetium Tc-99m sulfur colloid show a "hot spot" in the thorax *(arrow)*.

Anterior chest view **(C)** shows a central venous catheter, the tip of which is "hot" and is in the right atrium *(arrows)*.

The activity in the catheter indicates that the injection was made through the catheter, and there was adherence of the radioactive colloid in the tip of the catheter.

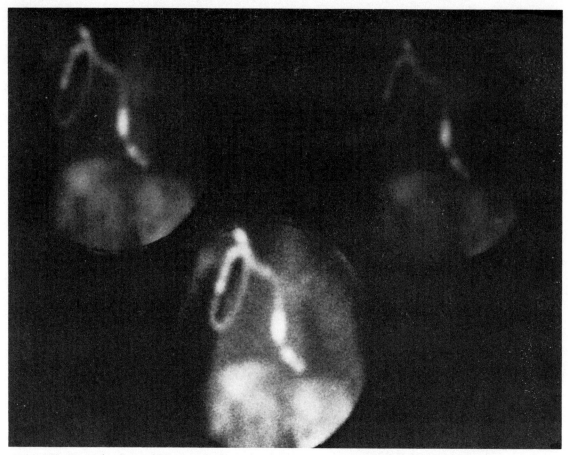

Case 9–16.—Tracing of a Central Venous Catheter by an Injection of a Radionuclide

During a process of cardiopulmonary resuscitation on a patient who was in hepatic failure and suffered cardiac arrest, a central venous catheter was inserted through the subclavian vein. However, the house staff was not confident that the catheter was in proper position, because there was high resistance to an attempt to draw blood back through the catheter. In order to trace the catheter, 2-mCi dose of technetium Tc-99m sulfur colloid was injected through the catheter and demonstrated that the tip of the catheter was in the right ventricle. Subsequently, a liver and spleen scan was obtained.

This is a very simple technique to demonstrate location and trace of an intravenous catheter and can be used in a patient who requires a radionuclide scan for any organ.

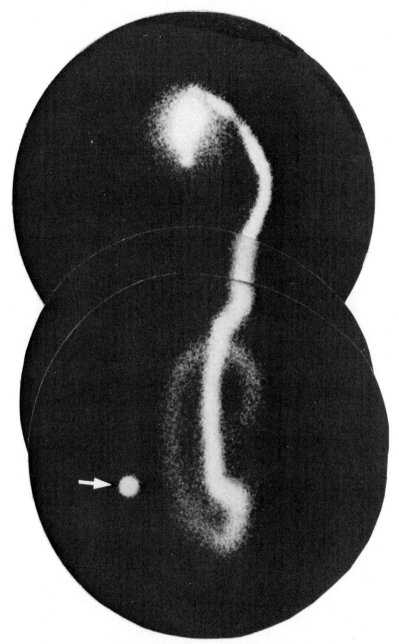

Case 9–17.—Misplaced Tip of a Ventriculoperitoneal Shunt Tube; Demonstrated on a Radionuclide Shuntogram
    Radionuclide ventriculoperitoneal shuntogram was obtained using technetium Tc-99m sulfur colloid on a 79-year-old woman who had a ventriculoperitoneal shunt operation because of her left frontal porencephalic cyst three years earlier. She was known to have a persistent left pleural effusion.
    The injection of the dose was made into the ventricle, left side, and the dynamic flow images were taken.
    A composite image of the radionuclide shuntogram shows the shunt tube that is curved at the diaphragm, runs upward and then downward; thus, most of the tube is in the left pleural cavity, making a ventriculopleural shunt.
    A hot marker (arrow) is placed over the xyphoid process.
    This is another example of effective tracing of an in vivo catheter or a tubing.

10

The Skeletal System

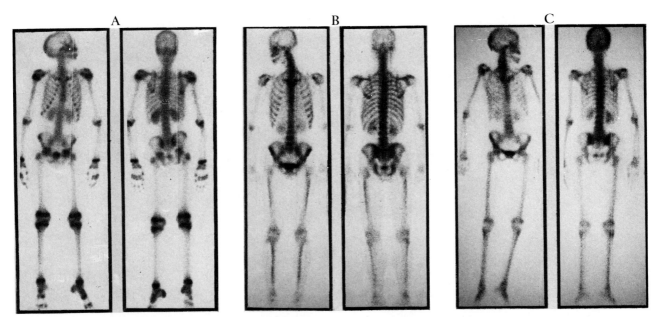

Case 10–1.—Normal Bone Scan in Different Age Groups; Young, Matured, and Older Man

Anterior and posterior views of whole body bone scans obtained using technetium Tc-99m medronate disodium on a 12-year-old boy **(A)**, 45-year-old man **(B)**, and on 74-year-old man **(C)**.

In all cases, the bone scan was normal. Characteristics of the bone scan findings are: intense uptake by the epiphyses and high costochondral junction uptake in young man; high uptake by the axial and long bones in matured man; and poor bony uptake in general and irregular and increased uptake in the joints in older man.

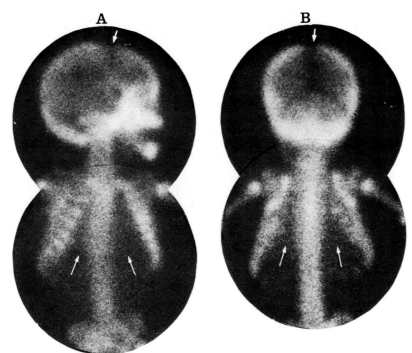

Case 10–2.—Infant Bone Scan

Composite images of anterior **(A)** and posterior **(B)** body bone scan obtained on a 2-month-old girl with suspected bone fractures using technetium Tc-99m medronate disodium. Noncalcified skull sutures make "broken skull" appearance *(small arrows)*. There is abnormally wide separation of ribs from the thoracic spine **(B)** and from the sternum **(A)** *(long arrows)*, because vertebral and costal cartilages are not completely ossified.

Poor resolution of the bones, sternum, and vertebrae indicates incomplete ossification of these bones as well.

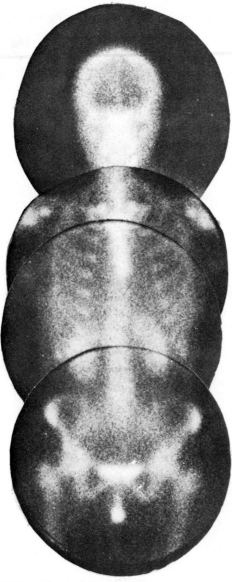

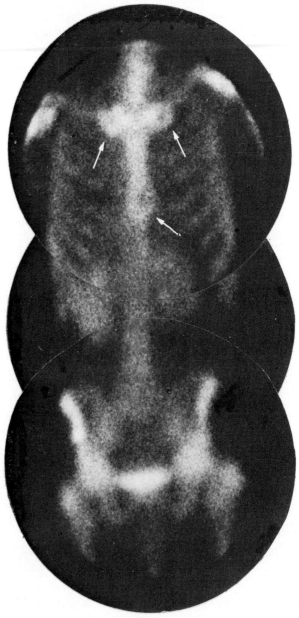

Case 10–3.—Hot and Small Sternum

Whole body bone scan on a 37-year-old woman with suspected breast carcinoma.

The anterior view body scan shows unusually small sternum with relatively increased uptake compared with other bones of thorax and pelvis. Such a small and hot sternum is not an uncommon variant on bone scans.

Case 10–4.—Prominent Sternoclavicular Junctions and Ballooned Distal Sternum

Bone scan, anterior view of the body, was obtained on a 47-year-old man with left shoulder and leg pain, using a 20-mCi dose of technetium Tc-99m medronate disodium. The scan shows ''bull's-eye'' changes in the bilateral sternoclavicular junctions and the distal sternum *(arrows).*

The ''balloon'' or ''bull's-eye'' in the distal sternum is a common variant. However, ''bull's-eye'' in the sternoclavicular junctions in addition to the distal sternum, forming a ''Picasso's sculpture,'' is a rare variant. A hot spot in the right iliac crest represents the site of prior bone marrow aspiration.

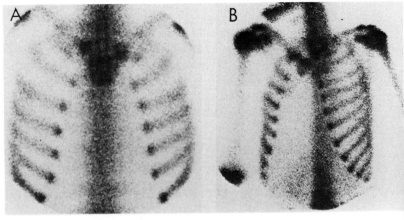

Case 10–5.—Absent Sternum on Bone Scan

A bone scan with technetium Tc-99m medronate disodium in a 12-year-old girl who has orbital rhabdomyosarcoma. Anterior (**A**) and oblique (**B**) views show no activity in the sternal segments exclusive of the manubrium, indicative of congenital lack of ossification of the sternum.

C, lateral radiography of the sternum shows no ossification of the sternal bodies exclusive of the manubrium.

(Courtesy of Mandell G.A., Heyman S. [Hospital of the University of Pennsylvania, Philadelphia]: Absent sternum on bone scan. *Clin. Nucl. Med.* 8:327, 1983.)

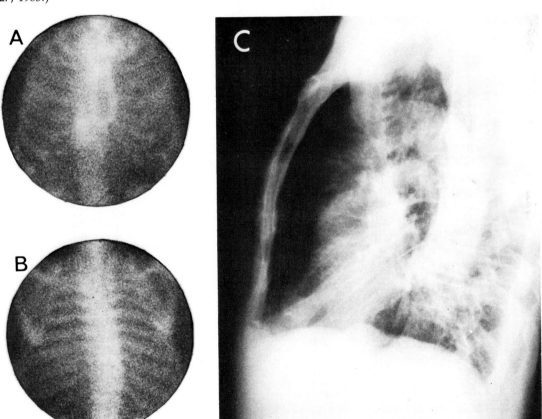

Case 10–6.—"Necktie Sign" on a Bone Scan

Anterior (**A**) and posterior (**B**) images of the bone over the chest were obtained on a 63-year-old man with known prostate carcinoma using technetium Tc-99m medronate disodium. The anterior view shows "empty" sternum causing a "necktie" sign. The lateral view chest radiography (**C**) shows normal sternum.

Such empty sternum is not a common variant; however, it may be seen more often in a patient with generalized osteoporosis.

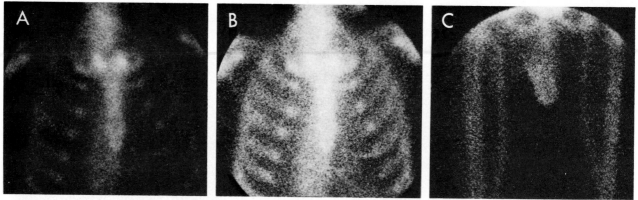

Case 10–7.—Prominent Sternoclavicular Joint With Absent Clavicle on a Bone Scan

Anterior camera view of chest bone scan (low- **(A)** and high- **(B)** intensity) obtained on a 78-year-old man using technetium Tc-99m medronate disodium shows hot sternoclavicular joint. Such high activity in the sternoclavicular joint is a relatively common finding in individuals without the joint abnormality.

The clavicles are not imaged on the scan. Nonvisualization of the normal clavicles is also a common finding on a bone scan.

Anterior upper thigh image **(C)** on the same patient shows clear images of the bilateral femoral arteries, another common finding on a bone scan of elderly individuals, indicating calcification of the arteries.

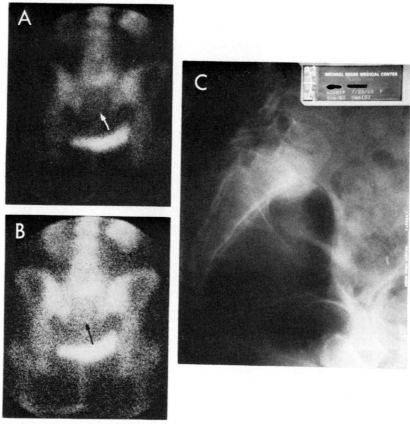

Case 10–8.—Nonvisualization of a Normal Sacrum on a Bone Scan

Posterior view pelvic bone scan **(A)** obtained on a 61-year-old woman with low back pain shows nonvisualization of the sacrum *(arrows)*. A high-intensity exposure of the same view **(B)** failed to show the sacrum. Radiograph of the sacrum **(C)**, however, shows no bony abnormality except a mild, generalized osteopenia.

Nonvisualization of a normal, auxiliary bone on a bone scan is not an infrequent finding in elderly patients.

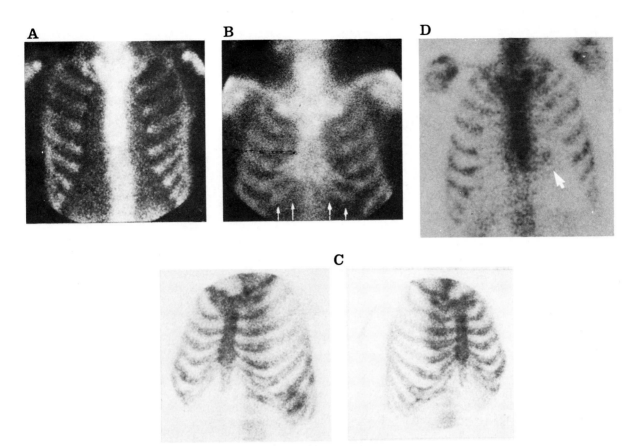

Case 10–9.—Various Degrees of Calcification of Costal Cartilage Demonstrated on a Bone Scan

Anterior chest view of a bone scan obtained using technetium Tc-99m medronate disodium on a 20-year-old woman shows a normal sternum and ribs **(A).** The costal cartilages are not imaged on the bone scan.

Another anterior chest bone scan on a 71-year-old man shows the costal cartilages with uptake almost equal to the ribs **(B,** *arrows*), indicating calcification of the cartilages. Such calcification of cartilages is a normal phenomenon in elderly individuals but can also be seen in younger patients with hyperostosis **(C).**

When there is unilateral uptake in the costal cartilage **(D,** *arrow*), the case should be carefully evaluated for possible myocardial infarction that may have caused localization of the bone-scanning agent.

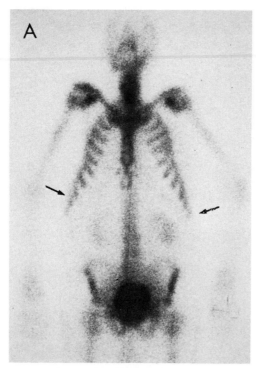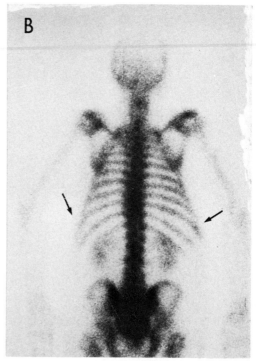

Case 10–10.—Barrel Chest Due to Emphysema Seen on a Bone Scan

Body bone scan was obtained using technetium Tc-99m medronate disodium on a 62-year-old man with a long history of chronic obstructive lung disease and recently discovered lung carcinoma.

The scan, anterior **(A)** and posterior **(B)** views, shows the lower rib margin to be flared outward *(arrows)*. On the posterior image, the ribs are horizontal and lower intercostal spaces are very wide.

The findings are characteristic chest conditions fixed in hyperinflated lungs seen in patients with advanced emphysema.

Case 10–11.—Elongated Skull and Asymmetrical Rib Images on a Bone Scan

Anterior view head and chest bone scan obtained using technetium Tc-99m medronate disodium on a 55-year-old woman with breast carcinoma shows unusually elongated skull with prominent orbit. An elongated or oval skull is not an unusual variant. In this case, however, the skull appears elongated because the patient had her chin down, making the shape of the skull appear to be more elongated on the scan. Shape of the facial bones and skull changes depends on the angle of the head view.

Anterior chest is asymmetrical, with ribs of the left chest imaged more clearly than the ribs of the right chest. The patient had undergone left radical mastectomy; thus, soft tissue attenuation is eliminated from the left chest and demonstrates left ribs better, while photon activity from the ribs of the right chest is attenuated by the chest wall muscles and the breast.

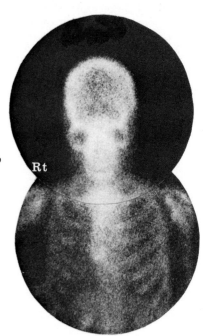

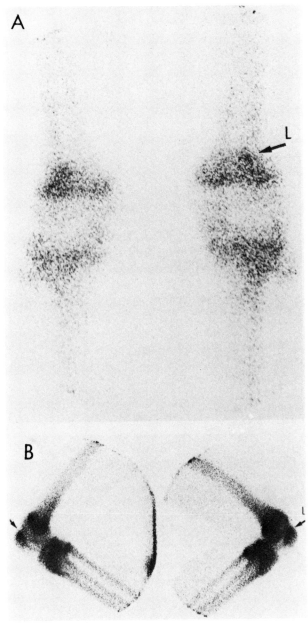

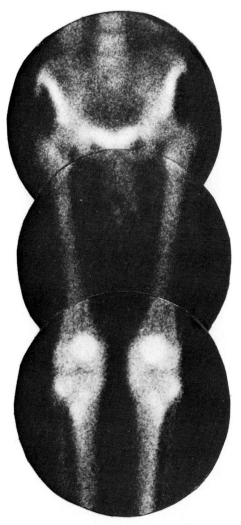

Case 10–12.—"Dorsal Defect" of the Patella on Radionuclide Bone Scan

Bone scans of the knees were obtained using technetium Tc-99m medronate disodium. The anterior view **(A)** shows some focal activity accumulating superiorly, especially on the left side *(arrow)*. Lateral views **(B)** demonstrate increased activity in the superior posterior aspect of the patella, the left greater than the right *(arrows)*.

The "dorsal defect" of the patella occurs in about 1% of the population, and the lesions are usually asymptomatic and bilateral in one-third of cases. The postulated etiology of the developmental defect is delayed ossification.

(Courtesy of Mandel G.A., Heyman S. [Hospital of the University of Pennsylvania, Philadelphia]: Dorsal defect of the patella on radionuclide bone scan. *Clin. Nucl. Med.* 8:380, 1983.)

Case 10–13.—"Hot Patella" on a Bone Scan

A bone scan over the anterior pelvis and legs obtained using technetium Tc-99m medronate disodium shows unusually increased uptake by the bilateral patella—"hot patella."

There are reported cases of degenerative arthritis, fracture, possible metastases, bursitis, and Paget's disease causing such "hot patella" (Kipper M.S., Alazraki N.P., Feiglin D.H.: The "hot" patella. *Clin. Nucl. Med.* 7:28, 1982). However, the "hot patella" is not an uncommon normal variant.

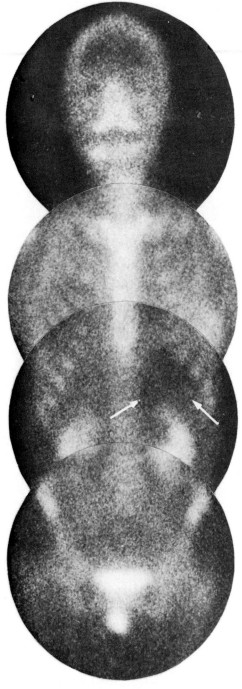

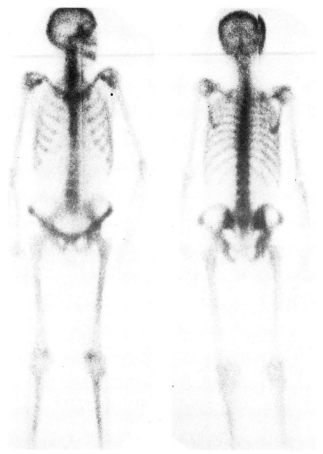

Case 10–15.—Superior-quality Bone Scan in a Patient With Chronic Renal Failure Who Received Hemodialysis After the Injection; Example Case 1

Anterior and posterior views of the whole body bone scan obtained using technetium Tc-99m medronate disodium on a 32-year-old man with chronic renal failure show superior quality of the scan with no soft tissue uptake. It is extremely unusual, however, to have nonvisualization of both kidneys and the urinary bladder on a good-quality bone scan. In a patient with diffuse metastatic disease involving entire axial skeleton and ribs, a bone scan may show excellent visualization of the bones and nonvisualization of the kidneys and soft tissue. In such a case, however, there is interskeletal shift of the activity. In a case of chronic renal failure a bone scan usually shows relatively high soft tissue uptake in addition to increased bone uptake (Cheng T.H., Holman B.L.: Increased skeletal: Renal uptake ratio, etiology, and characteristics. *Radiology* 136:455, 1980).

In the case shown here, patient received hemodialysis 85 minutes after the intravenous injection of the radiopharmaceutical, thus removing all free radionuclide from the circulation, leaving no radioactivity to be excreted through the renal system.

Case 10–14.—"Lunch Syndrome" on a Bone Scan

Composite image of an anterior bone scan obtained on a 62-year-old woman with history of right breast carcinoma shows a photon-deficient area in the left upper quadrant *(arrows)*, an artifact that appears frequently on bone scan and is called lunch syndrome (Croft B.Y., Teates C.D.: "Lunch syndrome," a bone-scanning artifact: Case report. *Clin. Nucl. Med.* 3:137, 1978), because it is the effect of photon attenuation by the food in the stomach.

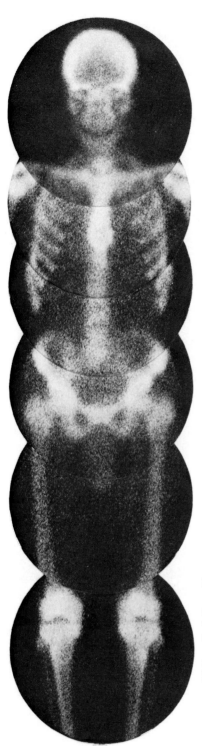
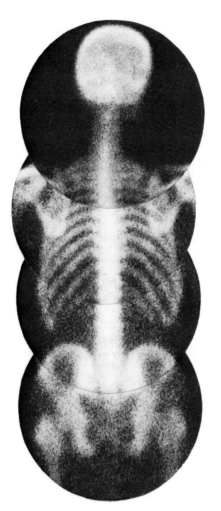

Case 10–16.—"Super Bone Scan" on a Patient With Chronic Renal Failure; Example Case 2

Composite image of the whole body bone scan, anterior and posterior view, obtained using technetium Tc-99m medronate disodium on a 47-year-old man with a seven-year history of renal failure shows excellent visualization of the skeletal system and nonvisualization of the kidney and bladder.

The patient did not receive hemodialysis after the injection. Increased skeletal uptake, "super scan," in this case, therefore, is attributable to secondary hyperparathyroidism—renal osteodystrophy.

Case 10–17.—Atrophy of Disuse Causing Falsely Increased Uptake in the Contralateral Normal Arm on a Bone Scan

Whole body bone scan was obtained using technetium Tc-99m medronate disodium, 3 mCi, on a 16-month-old girl with "left shoulder/arm pain" described by her mother. The scan showed diffusely increased uptake in the left humerus *(solid arrows)* compared with the right side *(open arrow)*.

The child had a history of "head trauma" six months before with subsequent right hemiparesis. Clinical evaluation failed to reveal evidence of injury in the right arm. The asymmetry of the uptake by the humerus was due to atrophy of disuse of the right arm.

Disproportionally larger head than trunk and larger upper body than lower body are normal features of a young child.

A "defect" seen in the left posterior temporal skull represents the photon attenuation by a hand that was holding the child's head.

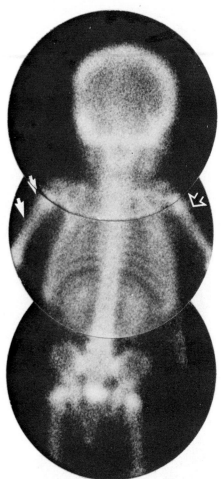

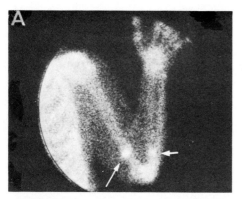 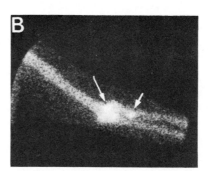 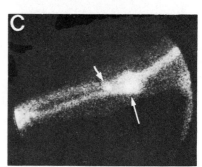

Case 10–18.—Site of Injections May Cause False Bone Lesions on Bone Scan

Anterior left arm view **(A)** of a bone scan obtained using technetium Tc-99m medronate disodium on a 66-year-old woman with a six-year history of breast carcinoma shows focal increased uptake in the humerus *(long arrow)* and between the radius and ulna *(short arrow)*.

When the arm was stretched, the "lesion of humerus" moved down to the elbow. The second lesion also moved to the proximal radius on the anterior image **(B)** and back to the soft tissue between the two bones on posterior view **(C)**. The foci of uptake corresponded to two injection sites.

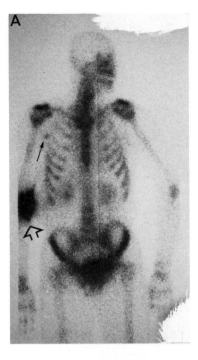

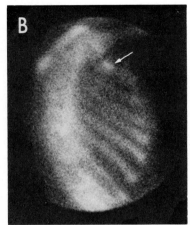

Case 10–19.—Visualization of Lymph Node on Bone Scan

Selective views, anterior **(A)**, and right lateral **(B)** images, of a whole body bone scan performed on a 32-year-old jogger for an evaluation of possible stress fracture shows a small focus of uptake in the right axillary region *(thin arrow)*. On the right lateral view the focal uptake was superimposed on a rib, causing an artifactitious lesion *(arrow)*.

A large area of intense activity seen on the right antecubital region indicates subcutaneous infiltration of the radiopharmaceutical *(open arrow)*. Imaging of the lymph nodes after subcutaneous injection of a bone-imaging radiopharmaceutical is a common phenomenon that may cause false positive bone scan interpretations.

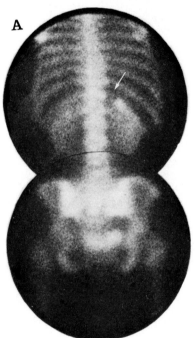

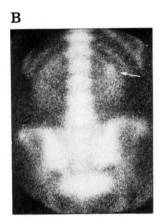

Case 10–20.—Artifactitious Abscission of a Rib Caused by a Hot Renal Calix on a Bone Scan

Posterior view bone scan at supine position **(A)** obtained using technetium Tc-99m medronate disodium on a 38-year-old woman with history of breast carcinoma shows an abscission of a right posterior 11th rib *(arrow)*. A repeated scan taken at upright position **(B)** shows a "hot calix" in the superior right kidney which now is located at the 12th rib level *(arrow)*. The abscission of the 11th rib is no longer demonstrated on the repeated scan.

The appearance of the "abscission" of the 11th rib was a visual illusion caused by the transverse process of the T-11 and the "hot calix"—dilated calix with retention of radionuclide—in the superior pole of the right kidney.

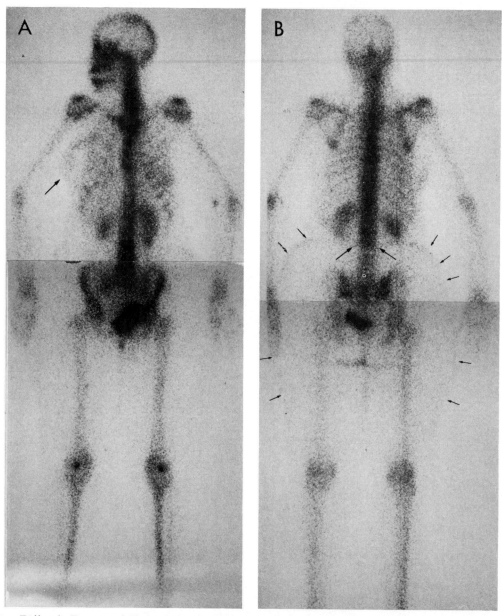

Case 10–21.—Diffusely Decreased Skeletal Uptake Due to Excessive Soft Tissue Attenuation Demonstrated on a Bone Scan

Anterior **(A)** and posterior **(B)** view whole body bone scan was obtained using technetium Tc-99m medronate disodium on a 54-year-old woman with history of breast carcinoma, right mastectomy, and an implant of right breast prosthesis. The anterior image shows a large rim activity with photopenic center on the right anterior chest **(A,** *arrow)*, demonstrating a breast prosthesis artifact. The posterior image shows diffusely decreased uptake in the lower lumbar spine, pelvic bones, and long bones of the extremities. The uptake by the spine shows a sudden change at the level of the 3rd lumbar spine **(B,** *long arrows)*.

The uptake by the upper lumbar spine and thoracic and cervical spine appears to be normal. There is a very large soft tissue mass in the shape of an elongated heart, its base coinciding with the 3rd lumbar spine level *(arrows)*. Excessive soft tissue mass in her lower body causes higher than usual tissue attenuation that is responsible for the decreased activity in the lower lumbar spine and posterior pelvic bones.

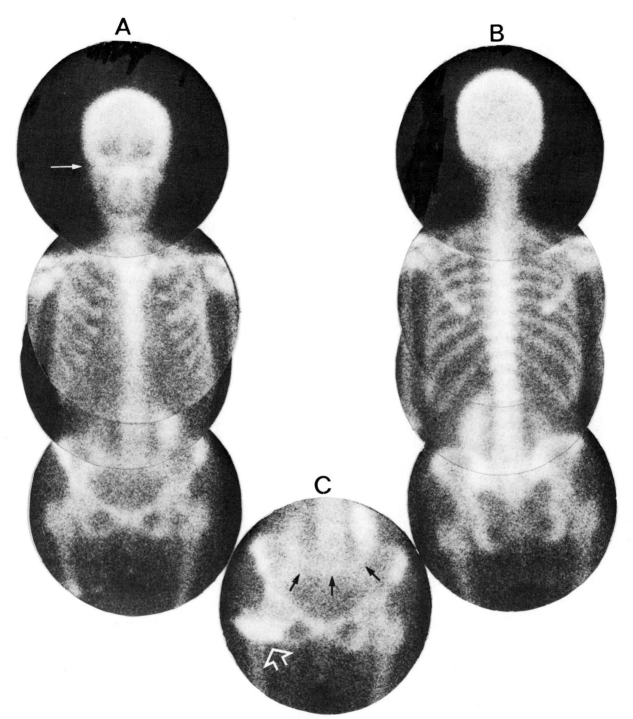

Case 10–22.—Horseshoe Kidney and Urine Bag Artifacts on a Bone Scan

Anterior **(A)** and posterior **(B)** bone images were obtained using technetium Tc-99m medronate disodium on a 63-year-old woman with lymphoma.

The supraorbital bone is not clearly imaged in this case; thus, the face view shows "eyes-closed" appearance *(white arrow)*.

The regional fine architecture and thickness of the skull varies very widely, and patterns of "normal distribution" of the radionuclide in the skull show more variation than any other part of the skeletal system.

Position of the kidneys is noted to be low, and a close-up pelvic view **(C)** shows the "horseshoe" kidney *(black arrows)*, which often cause falsely increased uptake in the sacroiliac joint and sacrum on posterior bone images. Also noted is a urinary bag lying in front of the hip, another common cause of bone scan artifact *(open arrow)*.

A

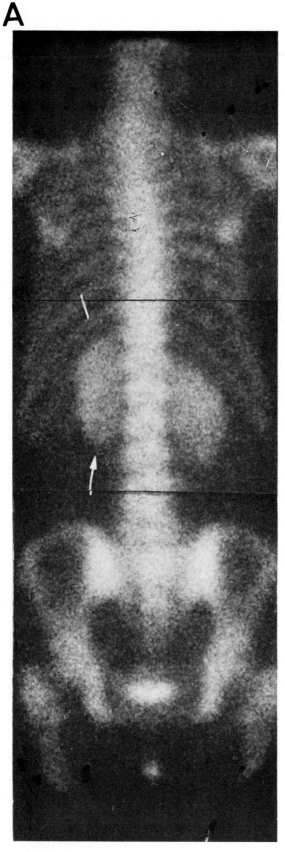

Case 10–23.—Kidney Clinging to the Vertebrae

Whole body bone scan was obtained on a 58-year-old woman with lung carcinoma and autoimmune hemolytic anemia, using technetium Tc-99m medronate disodium. The scan **(A)** showed the left kidney to be clung to the vertebrae *(white arrows)*. The liver and spleen scan **(B)** obtained on the same patient showed massive splenomegaly that displaced the kidney medially.

B

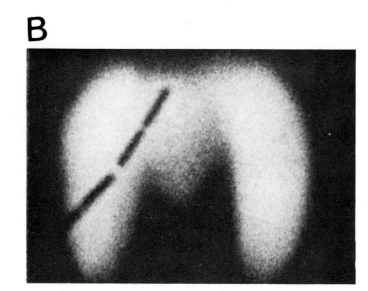

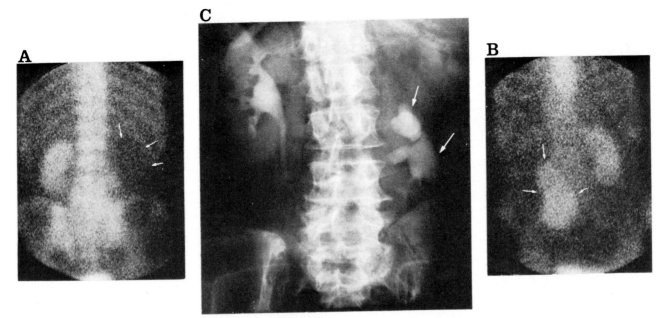

Case 10–24.—Malrotated, Ptotic Kidney on a Bone Scan

Posterior low back view, upright bone image **(A)** obtained using technetium Tc-99m medronate disodium on a 83-year-old woman shows low-lying left kidney and nonvisualization of the right kidney. The right renal bed appears to be photopenic *(arrows)*. Anterior pelvic image shows the right kidney in front of the right sacroiliac joint: a sacroiliac kidney *(?, arrow)*.

The intravenous pyelogram (IVP) **(C)**, however, shows malrotated (disrotation) right kidney with the renal pelvis directed laterally *(arrows)*, and the kidney is located above the pelvic cavity. These findings indicate that the right kidney is movable; therefore, it descends into the pelvis at upright position and ascends to the 3rd lumbar vertebra level at supine position. This causes discrepant positions of a movable kidney between IVP (supine) and renal or bone scan images (upright).

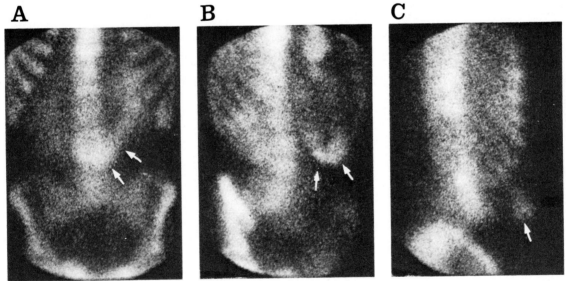

Case 10–25.—Demonstration of Laparotomy Scar on a Bone Scan

Camera views of bone scan were obtained on a 45-year-old woman with breast carcinoma using technetium Tc-99m medronate disodium.

An anterior image over the abdomen **(A)** shows abnormally increased uptake in the lumbar spine with extension to the left abdomen *(arrows)*. Right anterior oblique **(B)** and right lateral **(C)** views demonstrate the abnormal uptake to be in the anterior abdominal wall *(arrows)*. The patient had laparotomy for bilateral tubal ligation five months earlier, and the area of uptake corresponded to the well-healed laparotomy scar. Such uptake of bone scanning agent by healed surgical wound without radiological evidence of calcification has been reported (Siddiqui A.R., Stokka C.L.: Uptake of Tc-99m-methylene diphosphonate in a surgical scar. *Clin. Nucl. Med.* 5:274, 1980).

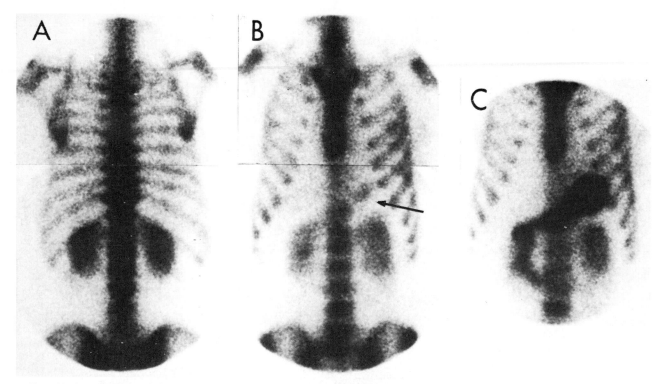

Case 10–26.—Radionuclide Activity in the Stomach Seen on a Bone Scan

Posterior **(A)** and anterior **(B)** body bone scan obtained using technetium Tc-99m medronate disodium on a 41-year-old woman with history of breast carcinoma shows an extraskeletal localization of radioactivity in the left upper quadrant **(B,** *arrow*).

Localization of the radioactivity was confirmed to be in the stomach by taking an anterior stomach image after a small, oral dose of technetium Tc-99m sulfur colloid **(C).** Plain radiograph showed no evidence of calcification of the stomach; therefore, the radioactivity in the stomach was presumed to be free sodium pertechnetate Tc-99m.

(Comments: localization of radioactivity in the stomach on a bone scan is a rare phenomenon. Early calcification of the stomach may not be detected on a plain radiograph.

Differentiation of free technetium Tc-99m activity in the stomach from the radioactivity localization in the stomach wall can be better made by giving a small amount of water, which will immediately dilute and wash away free technetium Tc-99m activity from the stomach.)

(Courtesy of William B. Martin, M.D., Division of Nuclear Medicine, Department of Radiology, University of Chicago Hospital, Chicago.)

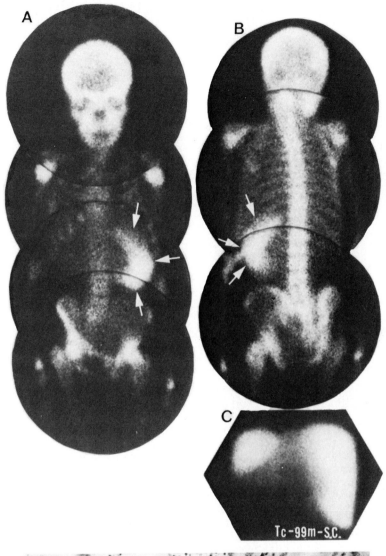

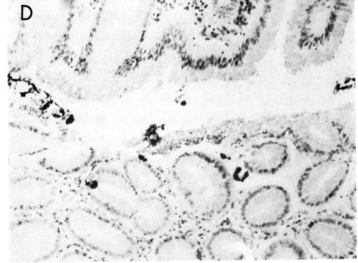

Case 10–27.—Localization of Bone-imaging agent in the Stomach

Whole body bone scan, anterior **(A)** and posterior **(B)** views, shows a diffusely increased uptake in the skull and facial bones. In addition, there is an abnormal soft tissue uptake in the stomach *(arrows)*. The kidneys are not visualized.

This scan was obtained on a 21-year-old black woman with sickle cell disease and chronic renal failure requiring hemodialysis for the past five years.

The increased uptake in the skull and nonvisualization of the kidneys are compatible with secondary hyperparathyroidism of the patient with renal failure. The uptake in the soft tissue was attributable to the localization of the bone-imaging agents in a spleen when there are ischemic changes or infarction, particularly in a patient with sickle cell anemia. In this case, however, the spleen image with technetium Tc-99m sulfur colloid **(C)** was normal, thus, the possibility of splenic infarction was ruled out.

The shape and location of the soft tissue uptake that showed no change on one-hour delayed images led to a conclusion: localization of the radionuclide in the calcified stomach. A plain radiograph of the abdomen failed to show calcification of the stomach, however.

Two months later, the patient suffered from an extensive pulmonary embolism and died of complications.

Histological examination of the stomach showed diffuse deposits of calcium in the mucous membrane (**C,** alizarin red S stain, ×420); precipitation of calcium ion in the gastric epithelium is facilitated by the excretion of acids, leading to local increase in hydroxyl ions forming calcium hydroxide and calcium hydroxyapatite crystal, and thus may cause increased concentration of the bone-imaging radionuclide.

(Comment: poor quality of the bone imaging agent, unbound free technetium Tc-99m, can be excreted through the salivary gland and stomach and cause imaging of the stomach. In such a case, however, the localization of the radioactivity can also be seen in the intestine.)

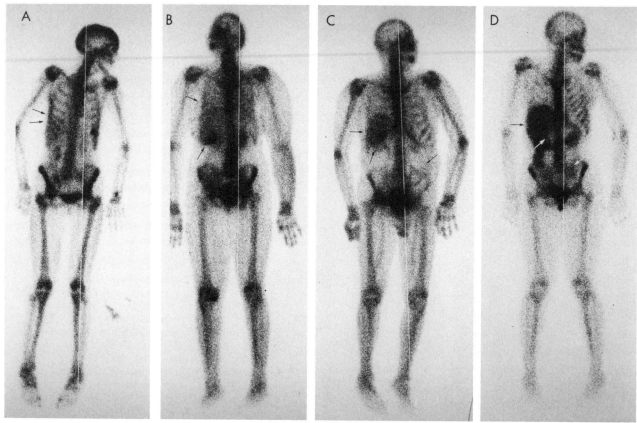

Case 10–28.—Visualization of the Normal Liver, Gallbladder, and Intestine on a Bone Scan; Artifacts Due to Poor Quality Control in Radiopharmaceuticals

Four example cases of anterior whole body bone scans obtained using technetium Tc-99m medronate disodium showing extraskeletal localization of the radionuclide in the gastrointestinal system.

A, an anterior image obtained 2.5 hours after the injection shows a faint image of the liver *(arrows)*. The patient had a liver scan performed 48 hours earlier, the most common cause of the visualization of the liver on a bone scan.

B, an anterior image obtained 3.5 hours after the injection shows visualization of the liver and intense activity in the gallbladder *(arrow)*. The localization in the gallbladder was confirmed by repeated images at various angles using a gamma camera. This patient did not have a recent radionuclide liver imaging procedure.

C and **D,** anterior view obtained 4.5 **(C)** and 5 **(D)** hours after the injection show the liver, the gallbladder, and intestine *(arrows)*.

(Comments: localization of the bone imaging agent in the liver, gallbladder, and intestine was reported by several investigators; however, the precise mechanism has not been documented (Zimmer A.M., Pavel D.G.: Experimental investigations of the possible causes of liver appearance during bone scanning. *Radiology* 126:813, 1978; and Conway J.J., Weiss S.C., Khentigan A., et al.: Gallbladder and bowel localization of bone imaging radiopharmaceuticals. *J. Nucl. Med.* 20:622, 1979). In none of our cases was the spleen imaged, thus the mechanism was not through a formation of colloid as suggested by others. The most plausible mechanism of such localization in the normal liver, gallbladder, and intestine is poorly controlled quality of the sodium pertechnetate Tc-99m generator and/or the eluate (Sherkow L, Fabich D., Ryo U.Y., et al.: Visualization of the liver, gallbladder and intestine on bone scintigraphy. *Clin. Nucl. Med.* in press).

Case 10–29.—Visualization of the Spleen on a Bone Scan

Anterior **(A)** and posterior **(B)** view bone images over the chest and abdomen obtained using technetium Tc-99m medronate disodium on a 12-year-old boy with sickle disease show prominent image of the spleen *(arrows)*. Such splenic uptake on a bone scan is a frequent finding in a patient with sickle cell disease and is reported to represent splenic infarction (Fischer K.C., Shapiro S., Treves S.: Visualization of the spleen with a bone-seeking radionuclide in a child with sickle-cell anemia. *Radiology* 122:398, 1977). There is another study, however, that indicates that the splenic uptake on a bone scan indicates ischemic changes but not infarction (Ryo U.Y., Kim I., Pinsky S.M.: Evaluation of splenic function in patients with sickle cell anemia. *Clin. Res.* 27:305, 1979).

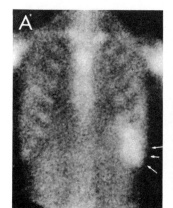
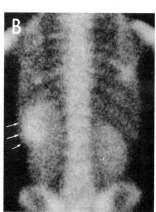

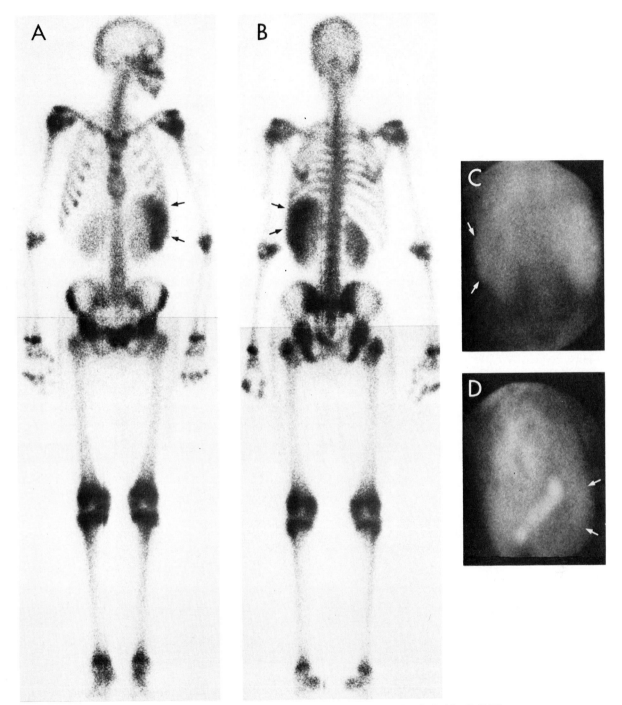

Case 10–30.—Prominent Image of the Spleen on a Bone Scan in a Patient With Sickle Cell Disease

Anterior **(A)** and posterior **(B)** views of whole body bone scan obtained using technetium Tc-99m medronate disodium on a 22-year-old man with sickle cell disease show a prominent image of an enlarged spleen *(arrows)*.

A liver and spleen scan obtained using technetium Tc-99m sulfur colloid failed to demonstrate the spleen, a finding consistent with functional asplenia and frequently seen in patients with sickle cell disease (Sain A., Sham R., Silver L.: Bone scan in sickle cell crisis. *Clin. Nucl. Med.* 3:85, 1978).

A posterior **(C)** and left lateral view **(D)** of the spleen taken using technetium Tc-99m-labeled red blood cells show the spleen; thus, an infarction of the spleen is ruled out.

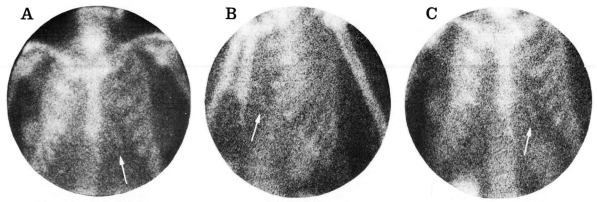

Case 10–31.—Incidental Finding of Myocardial Infarction on a Bone Scan

Anterior chest bone scan **(A)** obtained on a 74-year-old woman with history of breast carcinoma, three hours after an intravenous dose of technetium Tc-99m pyrophosphate shows a small area of extraskeletal uptake *(arrow)*. Direction of the linear uptake indicates that it is not a calcified costal cartilage. Because of the suspicious finding, the patient had repeated images taken.

Delayed left anterior oblique **(B)** and anterior views **(C)** obtained five hours after the injection again show the focal uptake in the region of the heart but with lesser intensity *(arrow)*. Such decreasing intensity supports that the uptake is in the ischemic myocardium.

The patient had an episode of severe chest pain five days earlier.

(Comments: when a focal uptake in the left chest in the region of the heart is noted on a bone scan, suspicion of a recent myocardial infarction must be raised though an old infarction may also cause such scan findings (Lyons K.P., Olson H.G., Brown W.T., et al.: Persistence of an abnormal pattern on ^{99m}Tc pyrophosphate myocardial scintigraphy following acute myocardial infarction. *Clin. Nucl. Med.* 1:253, 1976).

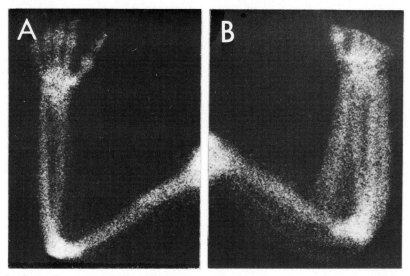

Case 10–32.—Lymphedema Demonstrated on Bone Scan

Right and left arm bone image obtained using technetium Tc-99m medronate disodium on a 73-year-old woman with history of left mastectomy show diffusely increased soft tissue uptake in the left arm **(B)**, while bone image of the right arm **(A)** is essentially normal.

As a complication of the left mastectomy, the patient developed lymphedema of the left entire arm that retained the radiopharmaceutical in the soft tissue, a not infrequent finding on a bone scan in a patient who underwent radical or modified radical mastectomy.

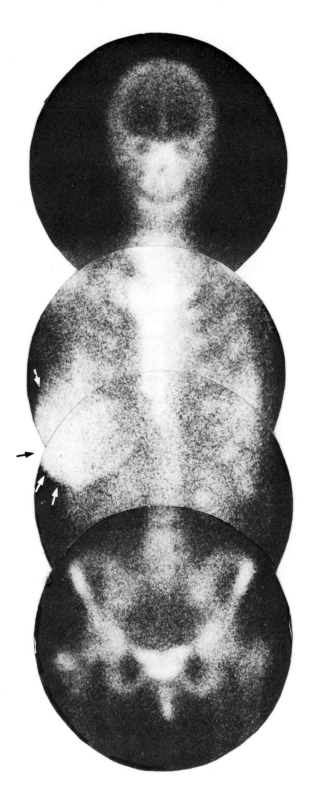

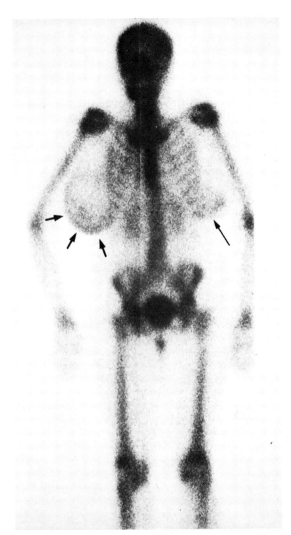

Case 10–34.—Asymmetrical Breast Uptake on Bone Scan

Anterior bone image obtained using technetium Tc-99m medronate disodium on a 44-year-old woman with recently found breast carcinoma shows diffuse uptake in the right entire breast *(arrows)*. There is focal uptake seen in the left breast *(long arrow)*.

She had palpable mass in the right breast that received a biopsy a week prior to the bone scan. The diffuse uptake represents inflammatory reaction secondary to the biopsy.

Asymmetry in the breast uptake, in most cases, indicates unilateral breast inflammation/infection or mass lesion.

Case 10–33.—Unilateral, Diffuse Breast Uptake on a Bone Scan

Composite image of an anterior bone scan obtained using technetium Tc-99m medronate disodium on a 34-year-old woman with history of breast carcinoma shows diffusely increased uptake by the right breast *(arrows)*.

The patient received left mastectomy and was taking birth control pills.

Such unilateral breast uptake on a bone scan is seen in patients who are lactating or taking birth control pills and had unilateral mastectomy, or who have recently undergone a breast biopsy, have unilateral mastitis, or extensive tumors in one breast.

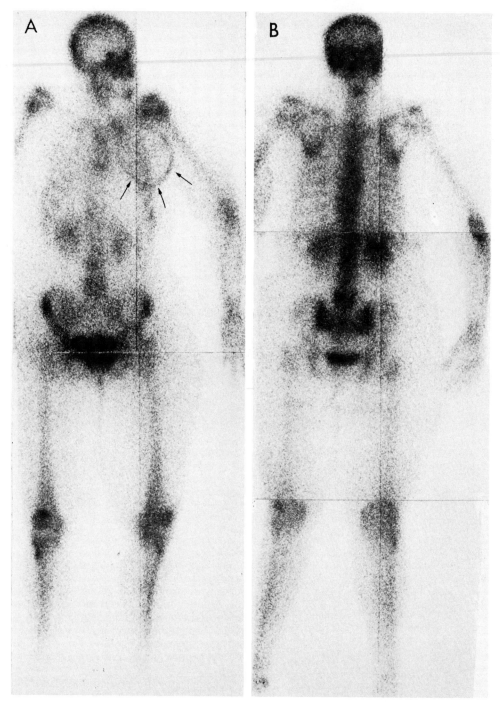

Case 10–35.—Visualization of a Breast Implant on a Bone Scan

Whole body bone scan was obtained using technetium Tc-99m medronate disodium on a 56-year-old woman with history of breast carcinoma. The scan, anterior **(A)** and posterior **(B)** images, shows a circle of activity in the left anterior chest *(arrows)*. This circle corresponded to the left breast implant performed one year ago, after the left mastectomy. The bone scan shows relatively poor uptake by the skeletal system. Such poor uptake despite good-quality radiopharmaceutical can be attributable to high soft tissue attenuation and soft tissue uptake in obese patients.

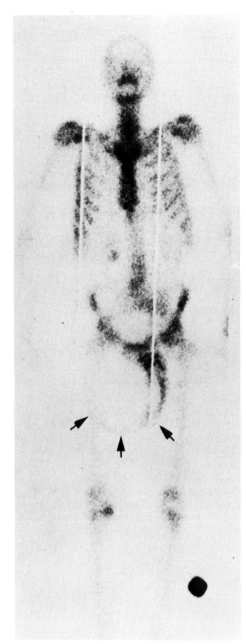

Case 10–36.—Unusual Soft Tissue Uptake in an Inguinal Hernia on a Bone Scan; Radiopharmaceutical Artifact

Anterior view whole body bone scan obtained using technetium Tc-99m medronate disodium shows a large "ring activity" below the pelvis *(arrows)*. The unusual uptake corresponded to a large right inguinal hernia.

Comments: another example case that emphasizes the importance of examining the patient before the conclusion of an imaging procedure and correlating unusual or abnormal findings with physical findings.

(Courtesy of Hussein M. Abdel-Dayem, M.D., Department of Radiology and Nuclear Medicine, Faculty of Medicine, Kuwait University, Safat, Kuwait.)

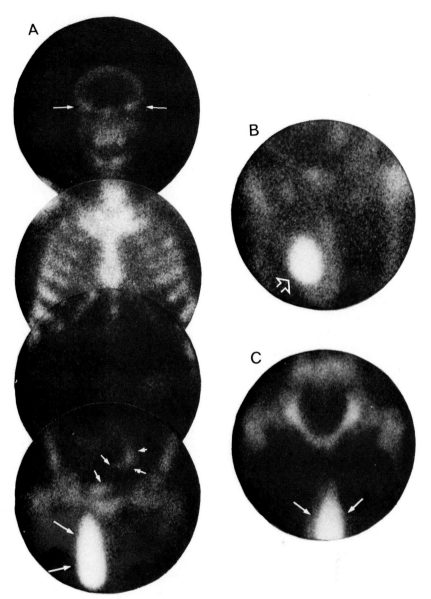

Case 10–37.—Scrotal Herniation of the Urinary Bladder Demonstrated on a Bone Scan

Whole body bone scan was obtained on a 69-year-old man with prostate carcinoma using technetium Tc-99m medronate disodium. The anterior body image **(A)** shows more prominent supraorbital bone uptake *(thin arrows)* than uptake by the zygomatics, causing "warrior image." The scan also shows calcified costal cartilage *(arrows)*, another common variant, particularly in elderly individuals.

Irregular areas of uptake seen in the pelvis *(small arrows)* represent the activity retention in dilated ureters that should not be interpreted as abnormal skeletal uptake.

A large, ovoidal area of intense activity is seen in the inguinal region *(arrows)*. A "SOC view" (sitting-on-collimator) **(C)** reveals that the "sac" with intense activity lies outside of the pelvic cavity *(arrows)*. The sac represented a scrotal herniation of the urinary bladder.

A repeated anterior pelvic image taken after a voiding and manual squeeze of the scrotal hernia **(B)** shows the shrunken sac *(open arrow)*. Herniation of the bladder is not an uncommon anomaly, especially in older people. One study reported 5 cases of scrotal hernia among 50 patients with herniation of the bladder (Liebeskind A.L., Elkin M., Goldman S.H.: Herniation of the bladder. *Radiology,* 106:257, 1973).

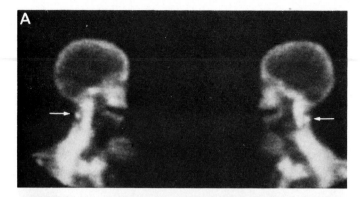

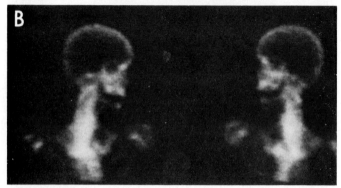

Case 10–39.—Gold Earring Causing Artifactitious Cervical Bone Lesions

Right and left lateral head and neck bone images **(A)** were obtained as a part of whole body bone scan using technetium Tc-99m medronate disodium on a 56-year-old woman with breast carcinoma. The scan shows small, isolated bone lesion in both sides of the upper cervical spine *(arrows).*

Photon-deficient rim surrounding the "bone lesion" indicates probable artifacts. The patient was wearing large, circular, gold earrings. The isolated bone lesions disappeared on repeated lateral views taken without the earrings **(B).**

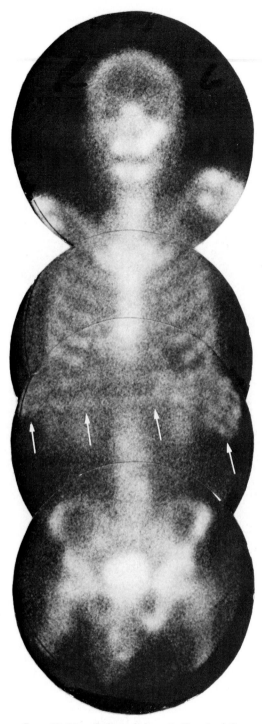

Case 10–38.—Splinted Arm in Front of the Abdomen; Artifact on a Bone Scan

Composite image of the body bone scan obtained with technetium Tc-99m medronate disodium shows the right forearm and hand in front of the abdomen *(arrows).* The patient had pathologic fracture of the right humerus, and the right arm was fixed (splinted) in front of his abdomen.

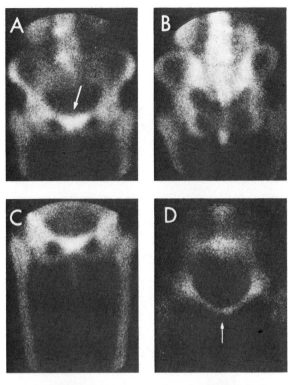

Case 10–40.—Osteitis Pubis or Residual Urine in the Bladder on a Bone Scan

Anterior pelvic bone scan **(A)** obtained using technetium Tc-99m medronate disodium shows intense activity in the symphysis pubis *(arrow)*. High activity in this region is usually attributed to a small amount of residual radioactive urine. Because of complex tissue attenuation, posterior pelvic view **(B)** is not usually helpful.

Repeated anterior pelvic view can easily be taken after a voiding. However, a small amount of residual urine cannot be voided completely; thus, osteitis pubis cannot be differentiated from the activity in a small residual urine on the basis of the scan finding alone.

An "SOC" view (sitting-on-collimator) often is useful on such an occasion. The SOC view shown here **(D)** is taken 18 hours after the bone scans so that no urinary activity is seen.

The symphysis pubis appears to be normal *(arrow)*; therefore, the activity seen on the earlier scans represented urinary activity.

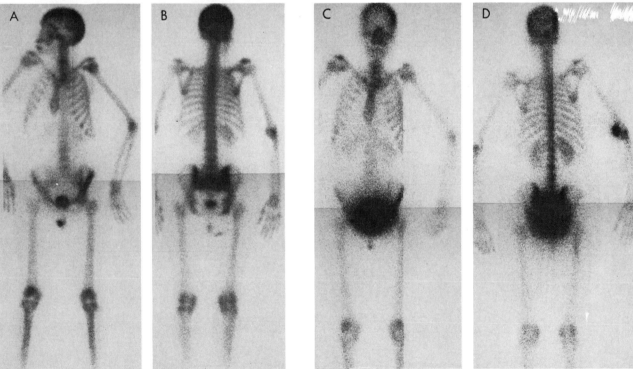

Case 10–41.—Decreased Uptake by the Skeletal System on a Bone Scan Caused by Oral Ingestion of Phosphate Compounds; Chemical-Radiopharmaceutical Artifact

Anterior **(A)** and posterior **(B)** views of a whole body bone scan was obtained using technetium Tc-99m medronate disodium on a 48-year-old woman with breast carcinoma metastasized to the liver and bones.

A follow-up bone scan obtained six months later **(C and D)** shows markedly diminished uptake by the skeletal system. The patient was receiving an experimental medication with an oral diphosphonate compound, Didronel, that is reported to be effective in strengthening the skeletal system and preventing or delaying lytic process in the bones.

Generally decreased skeletal uptake is attributable to the competition of unlabeled phosphate compound to the labeled radioactive molecules in adhering and binding to the surface of the bone, and excretion rate of the radiopharmaceutical is facilitated by the phosphate compound, a washout effect.

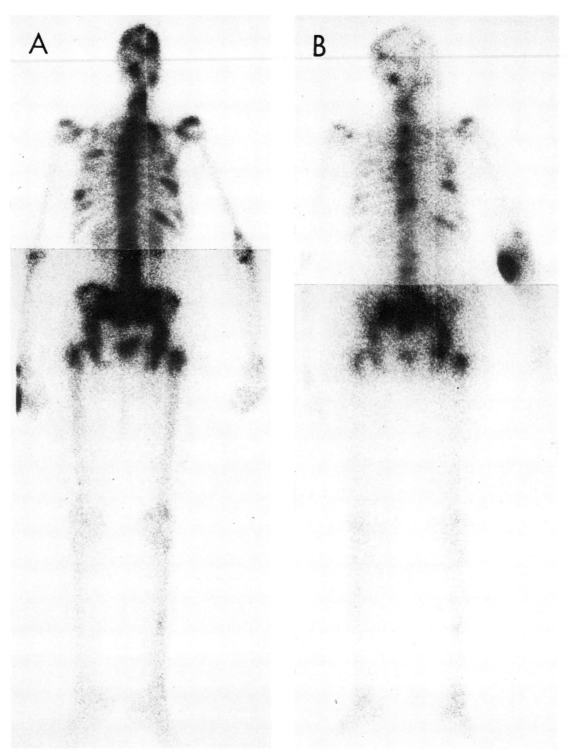

Case 10–42.—Effect of Increased Pool of Phosphate Compound on a Bone Scan; Another Example of Effect of Oral Phosphate Medication

Posterior view **(A)** whole body bone scan obtained using technetium Tc-99m medronate disodium on a 56-year-old woman with breast carcinoma shows extensive metastases. Abnormally small skull appearance is due to patient's movement. After the first pass over the left part of the whole body, she moved her head toward the left, a positional artifact.

A follow-up scan **(B)** obtained while the patient was receiving oral medication with the phosphate compound Didronel shows diffusely decreased uptake by the entire skeletal system. There is also decreased uptake by the metastatic lesions: chemical-radiopharmaceutical artifact.

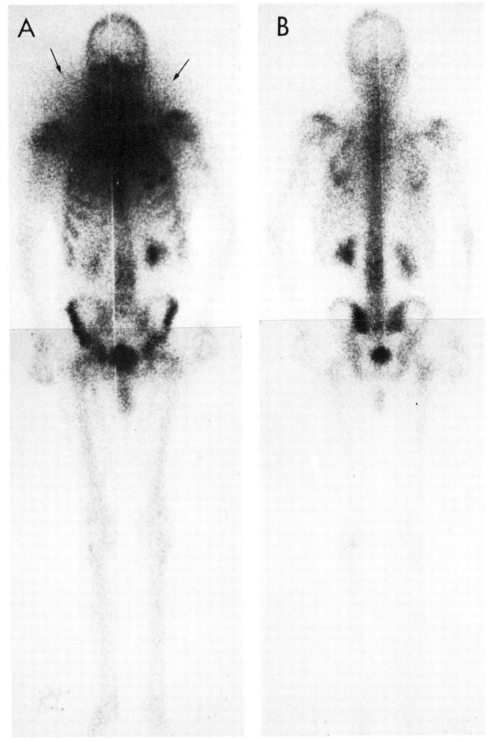

Case 10–43.—Effect of Higher-energy Radionuclide Contamination on the Quality of a Lower-Energy Radionuclide Imaging; Radiopharmaceutical and Technical Artifact

Anterior **(A)** and posterior **(B)** views of a whole body bone scan obtained using technetium Tc-99m medronate disodium on a 54-year-old man with bladder carcinoma shows an intense scatter photon activity in the anterior upper chest *(arrows)*. No radionuclide contamination could be identified. Radiospectroscopic study showed high sodium iodide I 131 activity in the thyroid. The patient had a "l-mCi dose of therapeutic iodine" a week ago at another hospital.

Comment: if the presence of sodium iodide I 131 in the thyroid is known in advance, a better bone image could be obtained by using medium-energy collimator, though the imaging time will be significantly prolonged.

(Courtesy of William B. Martin, M.D., Division of Nuclear Medicine, Department of Radiology, University of Chicago Hospital, Chicago.)

Case 10–44.—Increased Uptake in the Tibia Seen on a Pediatric Bone Scan Caused by Adherence of the Radionuclide in an Intravenous Catheter

Posterior view whole body bone scan obtained using technetium Tc-99m medronate disodium on a 3-month-old boy shows abnormally increased uptake in the medial left tibia *(arrows)*. Examination of the leg revealed an intravenous catheter in the distal saphenous vein through which the injection was made, causing the adherence of the radionuclide in the catheter. Such injection artifact from an injection of radionuclide through an intravenous catheter is a common problem, especially in the pediatric population.

(Courtesy of William B. Martin, M.D., Division of Nuclear Medicine, Department of Radiology, University of Chicago Hospital, Chicago.)

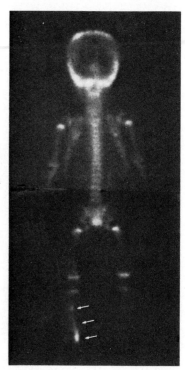

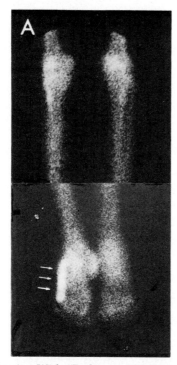

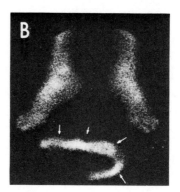

Case 10–45.—Contamination With "Radioactive Urine" on a Bone Scan; Example Case 1

Anterior bone image of the feet and lower legs **(A)** obtained as a part of whole body bone scan using technetium Tc-99m medronate disodium on an 84-year-old woman with lung carcinoma shows a linear, intense uptake in the lateral aspect of the right foot *(arrows)*. The uptake might cause a false impression of soft tissue and bone uptake. However, the linearity of the uptake and intensity suggest that more likely it is a contamination. When her slipper was taken off, there was no abnormal uptake in the foot **(B)**, and medial and posterior outline of the slipper was imaged due to the contaminaton with her "radioactive urine" **(B,** *arrows)*.

Since over 50% of the radionuclide is excreted through the renal system within two hours of the injection, a high radioactivity is expected in the urine. The most common artifact, therefore, in a bone scan is contamination with radioactive urine.

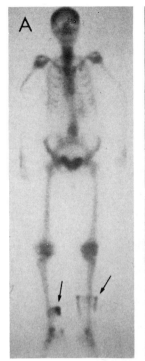
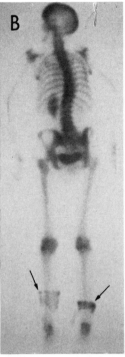

Case 10–46.—Contamination With "Radioactive Urine" on a Bone Scan; Example Case 2

Whole body bone scan, anterior **(A)** and posterior **(B)** views, obtained using technetium Tc-99m medronate disodium on a 64-year-old man with prostate carcinoma shows extraskeletal activity over the ankle and lower legs, creating a picture of a "man wearing a radioactive boot."

The patient had his socks contaminated with his radioactive urine.

(Courtesy of Robert L. Liebman, M.D., Department of Radiology, Westlake Hospital, Maywood, Ill.)

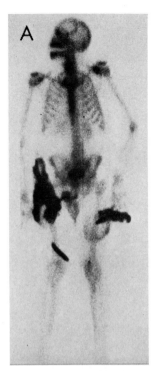
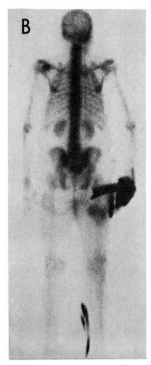

Case 10–47.—Contamination With "Radioactive Urine" on a Bone Scan; Example Case 3

Anterior **(A)** and posterior **(B)** views of a whole body bone scan obtained using technetium Tc-99m medronate disodium on a 67-year-old man with prostate carcinoma shows irregular areas of intense radioactivity over the lower half of the body. These intense activities are at different locations on the anterior image and on the posterior image. The patient was carrying a Foley catheter and a urine bag, which contained his "radioactive urine."

In a patient with a urine bag, the imaging technologist should be reminded to place the bag and tube outside of the bone-imaging field.

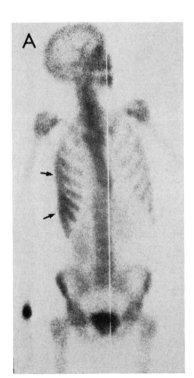
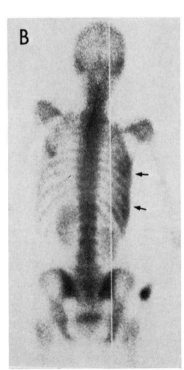

Case 10–48.—Radiation Osteitis of the Ribs on a Bone Scan

Anterior **(A)** and posterior **(B)** views of a body scan obtained using technetium Tc-99m medronate disodium on a 48-year-old woman with history of lung carcinoma shows diffusely increased uptake in the ribs of right anterior-lateral chest *(arrows)*.

The patient had received radiation therapy three months ago for a right lung carcinoma. The finding is a characteristic feature of radiation osteitis of the ribs. Such diffuse uptake in the unilateral thorax may represent malignant pleural effusion, though areas of increased uptake include intercostal spaces in case of pleural disease.

When a patient has collapsed lung with markedly narrowed intercostal spaces, differentiation of multiple rib uptake from pleural or pulmonary uptake may not be possible on a bone scan.

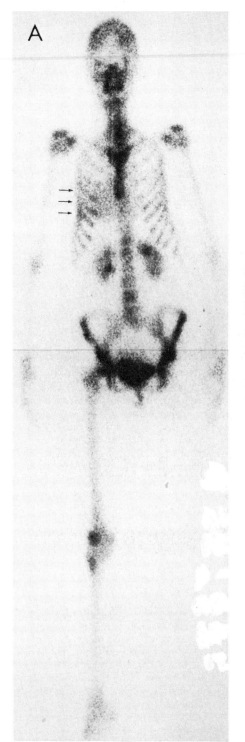

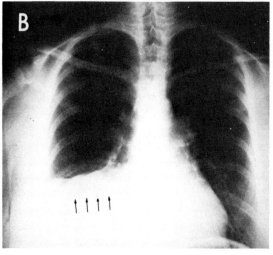

Case 10–49.—Localization of the Radionuclide in the Lung Demonstrated on a Bone Scan

Anterior view of a whole body bone scan obtained using technetium Tc-99m medronate disodium on a 40-year-old woman with history of liposarcoma and left leg amputation shows a diffuse activity in the right hemithorax (**A,** *arrows*). This area of diffuse uptake corresponded to a large infiltrate in the right lower lung (**B,** *arrows*). The lesion was later found to be a metastatic liposarcoma with foci of calcifications.

Numerous conditions are known to cause soft tissue localization of bone imaging agent, thus producing radiopharmaceutical artifacts on a bone scan (Heck L.L.: Extraosseous localization of phosphate bone agents. *Semin. Nucl. Med.* 10:311, 1980).

(Courtesy of William B. Martin, M.D., Division of Nuclear Medicine, Department of Radiology, University of Chicago, Chicago.)

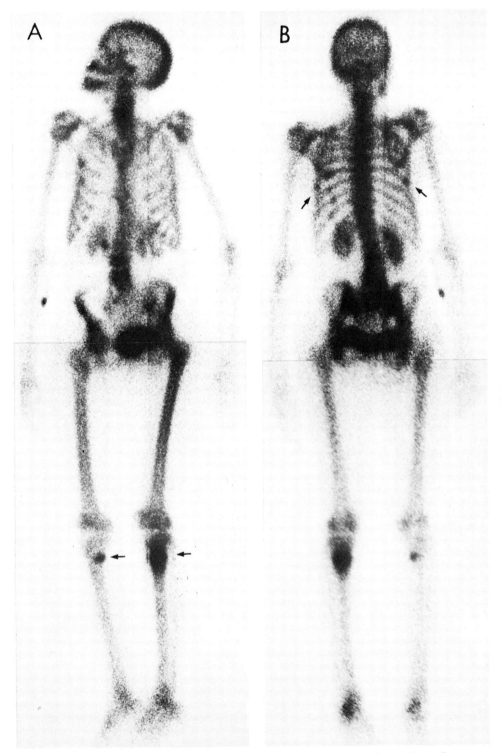

Case 10–50.—Postgastrectomy Osteomalacia With Pseudofractures Demonstrated on a Bone Scan

Anterior **(A)** and posterior **(B)** views of a whole body bone scan were obtained using technetium Tc-99m medronate disodium on a 78-year-old man who had undergone gastrectomy for carcinoma of the stomach and had been losing weight since. The scan shows markedly irregular uptake by the skeletal system and abnormally increased focal uptake in the tibia and in a few ribs *(arrows)*. Such focal areas of intense uptake might suggest metastases in a patient with known malignancy.

Bone radiograph revealed generalized osteomalacia with pseudofractures corresponding to the scan findings, typical features of malabsorption osteomalacia (Singh B.N., Spies S.M., Mehta S.P., et al.: Unusual bone scan presentation in osteomalacia: Symmetrical uptake—A suggestive sign. *Clin. Nucl. Med.* 3:292, 1978).

11

The Gallium Citrate Ga 67 Scan

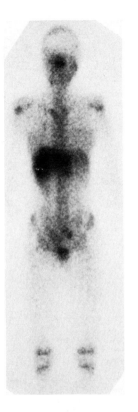
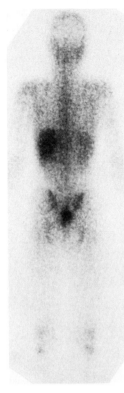

Case 11–1.—Normal Gallium Citrate Ga 67 Scan on a Child

Selective anterior **(left)** and posterior **(right)** planes of a tomographic gallium citrate Ga 67 scan obtained on a 10-year-old girl show normal distribution of the radionuclide in the liver, bone/bone marrow, breast, nasopharynx, and urinary bladder.

Characteristics of Ga 67 scan findings in a child are high activity in the epiphyses and less frequent visualization of intestinal Ga 67 activity.

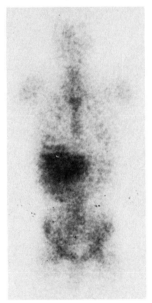
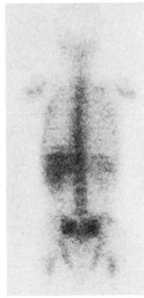

Case 11–2.—Normal Gallium Citrate Ga 67 Scan on an Adult Man

Selective anterior **(left)** and posterior **(right)** planes of a tomographic gallium citrate Ga 67 scan obtained on an adult man.

Highest activity distribution is in the liver, and second highest activity is in the bone/bone marrow. Faint activity distribution is seen in the spleen and nasopharynx. Lacrimal glands and salivary glands are almost invisible; normal variant.

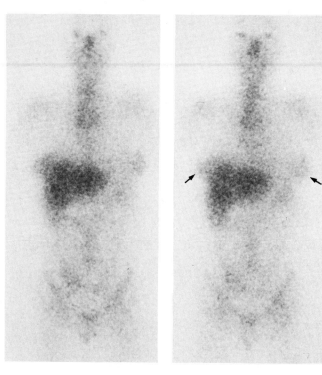

Case 11–3.—Normal Gallium Citrate Ga 67 Scan on a Woman

Selective anterior planes of tomographic gallium citrate Ga 67 scan on a nonlactating woman show a normal distribution of the radionuclide in the liver, bones, lacrimal glands, pharynx, and intestine. In addition, a symmetrical, mild uptake is seen in the breast *(arrows)*.

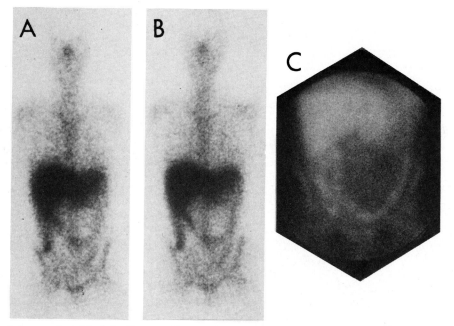

Case 11–4.—Usefulness of an Upright Gamma Camera Image of the Abdomen to Confirm the Intestinal Activity on a Gallium Citrate Ga 67 Scan

Selective anterior slices of tomographic gallium citrate Ga 67 scan obtained on a 22-year-old woman with history of lymphoma show curvilinear activity in the abdomen **(A and B)**, indicating that the activity represents Ga 67 in the large intestine. A repeated anterior image of the abdomen obtained at upright position using a gamma camera **(C)** shows clearer image of the ascending, hepatic flexure, and transverse colon. The entire colon is shifted downward on the upright camera view. Additional camera view of the abdomen often is useful to confirm the intestinal activity through a better resolution of the image and demonstration of the mobility of the intestine.

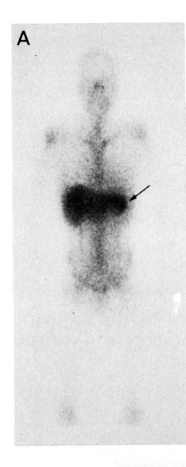

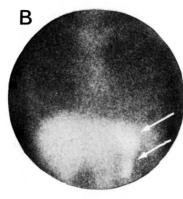

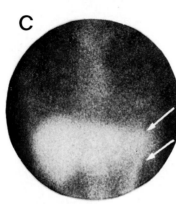

Case 11–5.—"Coke Test" to Confirm Localization of Gallium Citrate Ga 67 in the Stomach

Whole body tomographic scan was obtained using a 6-mCi dose of gallium citrate Ga 67 on a 23-year-old man who has congestive heart failure due to myocardiopathy and is clinically suspected to have endocarditis. A selective anterior tomographic image **(A)** shows diffuse uptake by the heart and focal, intense uptake in the left upper quadrant *(arrow)*. A close-up camera image **(B)** confirms the area with the unusual uptake *(white arrows)*. A repeated anterior image taken after a glass of carbonated soft drink (Coke) shows that the area of Ga 67 uptake became larger with diminished intensity **(C,** *arrows)*.

Such Ga 67 localization in the stomach has been observed frequently in patients with no known disease of the stomach.

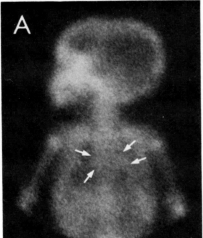

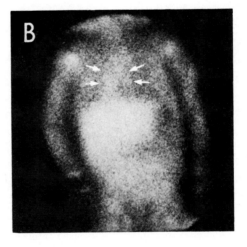

Case 11–6.—Two Example Cases of Thymus Uptake on a Gallium Citrate Ga 67 Scan

Anterior camera images of gallium citrate Ga 67 scan obtained on 1-year-old girl **(A)** and a boy **(B)** with suspected infectious disease show increased uptake in the upper mediastinum corresponding to the thymus gland *(arrows)*.

Such visualization of the thymus on Ga 67 scan of a young child (up to 5 years of age in our experience) is a normal finding.

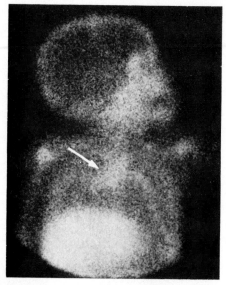

Case 11–7.—Image of the Thymus Gland on a Gallium Citrate Ga 67 Scan; Another Example

Anterior camera image of a gallium citrate Ga 67 scan obtained on a 2-year-old boy shows normal distribution of the radionuclide in the liver, skull, facial bones, epiphyses of humeri, and chest.

A prominent uptake is noted in the normal thymus gland *(arrow)*..

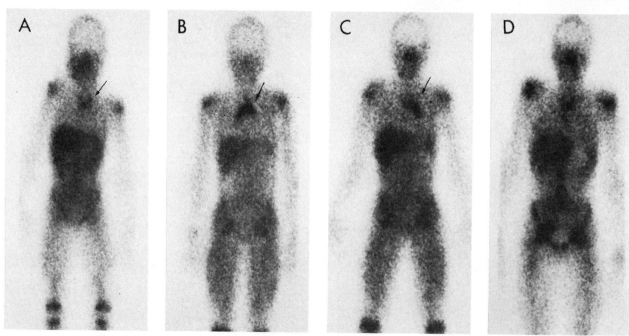

Case 11–8.—Image of a Normal Thymus Gland of an 8-year-old Boy on Gallium Citrate Ga 67 Scan

Selective anterior slice of tomographic gallium citrate Ga 67 scan obtained on a 5-year-old boy with biopsy-proved lymphoma **(A)** shows faint image of the thymus gland *(arrow)*. A follow-up Ga 67 scan, an anterior slice **(B)**, obtained two years later (at age 7) while he was receiving chemotherapy shows intense uptake by the apparently enlarged thymus *(arrow)*. The liver is smaller with decreased uptake.

Another follow-up scan obtained one year later (at age 8) showed obviously asymmetrical uptake in the left upper mediastinum **(C,** *arrow)*. In addition, abnormal uptake recurred in the right submandibular region. The patient underwent an excisional biopsy, and the left upper mediastinal uptake represented the thymus gland. The entire thymus gland was removed, and histological study of the gland was reported as essentially normal.

A follow-up Ga 67 scan obtained two years after the surgery (at age 10) **(D)** showed no abnormality.

(Comment: intense Ga 67 uptake by the thymus in the patient at age 7 **(B)** and 8 **(C)** was accompanied by relatively decreased liver and bone marrow uptake. These findings are all attributed to the chemotherapy. Mechanism of such enhanced Ga 67 uptake by the thymus is not clear; however, there is a report showing an intense Ga 67 uptake by a hyperplastic lymph node [Wahner H.W., Goellner J.R., Hoagland H.C.: Giant lymph node hyperplasia resembling abdominal abscess on gallium scan. *Clin. Nucl. Med.* 3:19, 1978].)

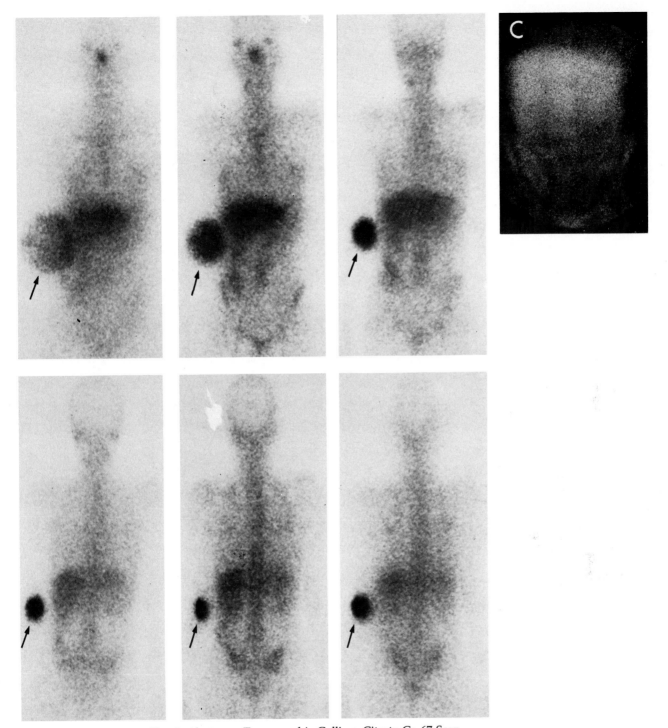

Case 11–9.—Injection Site Artifact on a Tomographic Gallium Citrate Ga 67 Scan
Selective anterior planes **(top row)** and posterior planes **(bottom row)** of tomographic gallium citrate Ga 67 scan show an intense activity at the injection site, extravasation of the Ga 67 *(arrows)* that interferes with the proper evaluation of the anterior right lobe of the liver.

A repeated anterior image of the liver taken with a gamma camera **(C)** shows a normal liver.

On the anterior planes of the Ga 67 images, the area with the infiltration of the Ga 67 appears to be very large, larger as the plane is farther away from the focused plane; out-of-focus artifact.

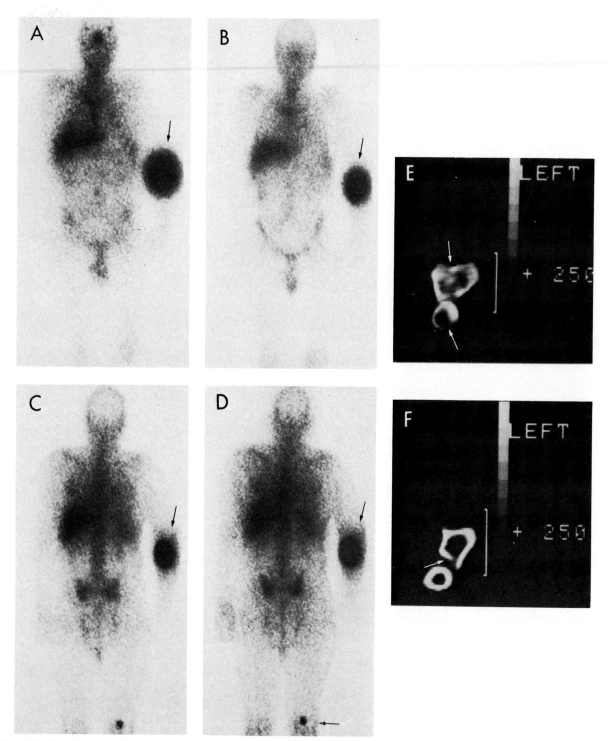

Case 11–10.—Increased Uptake in an Antecubital Fossa Due to Malignant Tumor Mimics an Injection Artifact on a Gallium Citrate Ga 67 Scan

Selective anterior slices (**A** and **B**) and posterior slices (**C** and **D**) of whole body tomographic gallium citrate Ga 67 scan obtained on a 49-year-old man show intense Ga 67 activity in the left elbow *(arrows)*. The finding is similar to an injection artifact (Case 11–9). The injection site, however, was recorded as the right arm. The patient had a painful and swollen left elbow. A computerized axial tomography (**E** and **F**) shows destructive bone lesion involving ulna and radius *(arrows)* that was later confirmed to be rhabdomyosarcoma. There was remote metastasis in the left popliteal region (**D**, *arrow*).

(Comments: radiopharmaceutical injection artifact, intense activity in the injection site, is a very common artifact seen on a bone scan or gallium citrate Ga 67 scan. Occasionally, however, a lesion may mimic injection artifact or vice versa. Therefore, it is very important to record and check site of injection in every case at the time of a scan interpretation.)

(Courtesy of W.B. Martin, M.D., Division of Nuclear Medicine, Department of Radiology, University of Chicago Hospital, Chicago.)

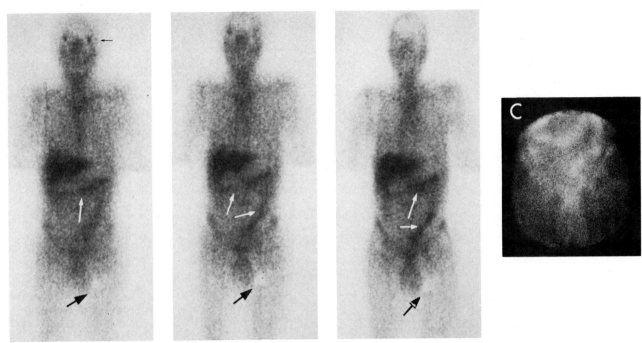

Case 11–11.—Attenuation of Photons by "Key-holder" on a Gallium Citrate Ga 67 Scan

Selective anterior planes of a tomographic gallium citrate Ga 67 scan obtained on a 65-year-old man with a mass lesion in the lung show a photopenic area in the medial thigh *(arrow)*. A repeated anterior image over the proximal thigh was taken after a key-holder and coins were removed from a pocket **(C)** and shows no attenuation artifact.

Prevention of such attenuation artifact on a Ga 67 scan is important because such an artifact may interfere with visualization of Ga 67-positive nodes.

The tomogram also shows a normal Ga 67 uptake by the lacrimal glands *(small black arrow)* and excretion of the radionuclide through the intestinal tract *(white arrow)*.

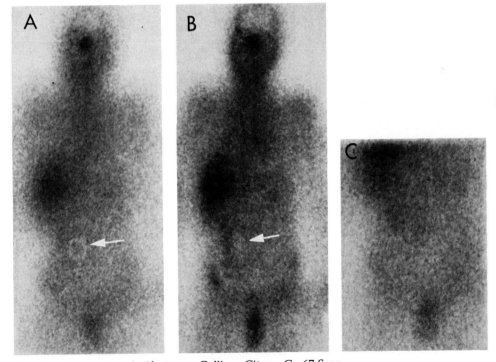

Case 11–12.—Photon Attenuation Artifact on a Gallium Citrate Ga 67 Scan

Selective anterior planes of tomographic gallium citrate Ga 67 scan **(A** and **B)** show no abnormal localization of the radionuclide.

There is a round rim of photon-deficient area in the abdomen *(arrow)*; photon attenuation by a belt buckle.

A repeated scan was obtained on the next day, after the belt buckle was removed **(C)**.

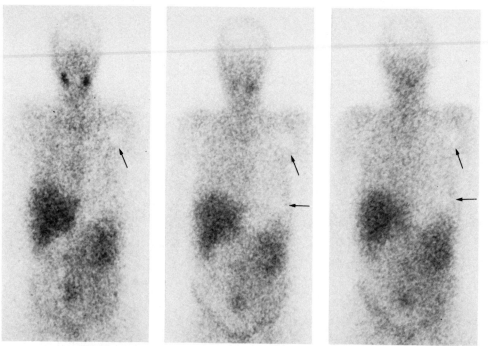

Case 11–13.—Pacemaker Artifacts on a Gallium Citrate Ga 67 Scan
Selective anterior planes of a tomographic gallium citrate Ga 67 scan obtained on a 74-year-old man with suspected malignancy show two photon-deficient areas in the left chest *(arrows)*. These two defects represented two cardiac pacemakers implanted in the chest wall.
The images also show unusually large thoracic cage with downward displacement of the liver, a common finding in patients with pulmonary emphysema.

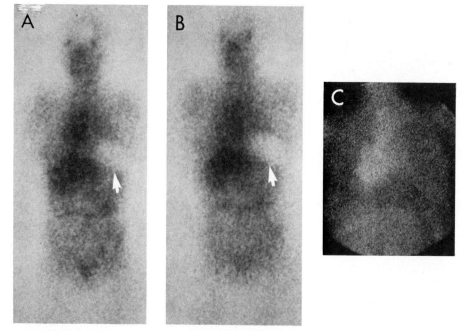

Case 11–14.—Artifact by Breast Prosthesis on a Gallium Citrate Ga 67 Scan
Selective anterior planes of tomographic gallium citrate Ga 67 scan obtained on a 60-year-old woman with history of breast carcinoma show a large photon-deficient area in the left thorax *(arrow)*.
The patient had a left mastectomy 11 years ago and was wearing a left breast prosthesis.
A repeated camera image **(C)** without the prosthesis shows normal left thorax. The patient was found to have extensive metastases in the right lung hilar nodes.

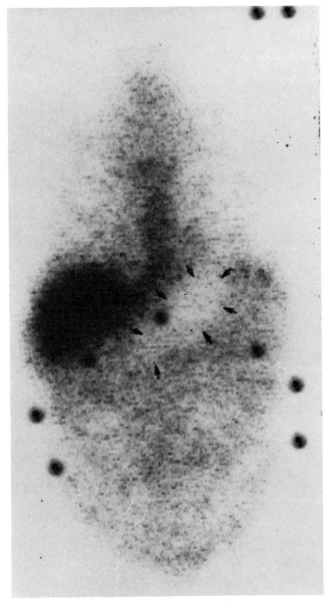

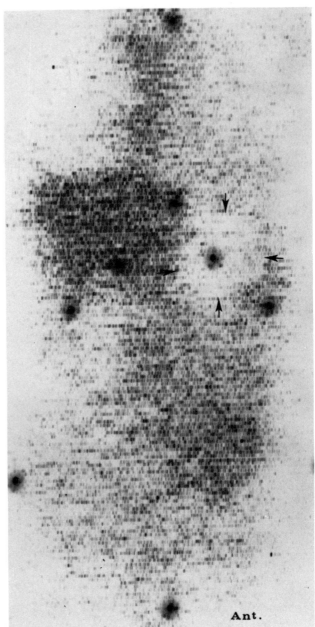

Ant.

Case 11–15.—"Lunch Sign" on an Indium In 111 Chloride Scan

An anterior view body image taken 72 hours after an intravenous dose of 3 mCi of indium In 111 chloride for an evaluation of bone marrows.

The image shows a large photon-deficient area in the epigastric region *(arrows)*, representing the full stomach.

Comment: the "lunch sign" is a common finding on a bone scan with technetium Tc-99m indium compound. With a higher-energy radionuclide, such as indium In 111 247 keV, such attenuation effect by food on a scan is a less common phenomenon. However, an unsually heavy, solid meal can cause such prominent attenuation, since 6-cm thick water can attenuate half of the 300-keV photon energy. The lunch sign should be differentiated from a large cystic lesion such as pancreatic pseudocyst. A repeated image taken a few hours later or on the next day should prevent the probable misinterpretation.

(Courtesy of Hussein M. Abdel-Dayem, M.D., Professor, Department of Radiology and Nuclear Medicine, Faculty of Medicine, Kuwait University, Safat, Kuwait.)

Case 11–16.—"Lunch Sign" on a Gallium Citrate Ga 67 Scan

Anterior view body scan obtained 72 hours after an intravenous dose of 3 mCi of gallium citrate Ga 67 using a rectilinear scanner shows a large photon-deficient area in the epigastric region *(arrows)*, representing the full stomach.

Such prominent "lunch sign" may be caused by heavy meal, or solid meal (Case 11–15). The use of rectilinear scanner with focused collimator enhances the appearance.

(Courtesy of Hussein M. Abdel-Dayem, M.D., Department of Radiology and Nuclear Medicine, Faculty of Medicine, Kuwait University, Safat, Kuwait.)

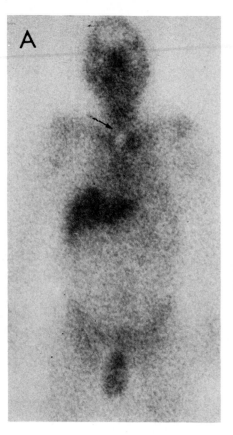

A

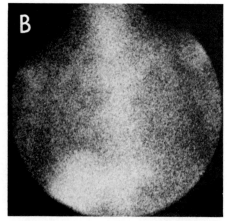

B

Case 11–17.—Necklace Pendant Artifact on a Gallium Citrate Ga 67 Scan

Selective anterior plane **(A)** of a tomographic gallium citrate Ga 67 scan shows a round photon-deficient area in the suprasternal region *(arrow)*. The patient was wearing a gold pendant. A repeated chest view obtained with gamma camera **(B)** after the pendant was taken off shows no more attenuation artifact.

A thorough bowel preparation can yield clean abdomen without intestinal activity on a Ga 67 scan **(A)**.

Case 11–18.—Tracheotomy Wound on a Gallium Citrate Ga 67 Scan

Selective anterior planes of a tomographic gallium citrate Ga 67 scan obtained on a 53-year-old woman show abnormal uptake in the anterior neck *(arrow)*. This abnormal uptake corresponded to her tracheostomy wound. Though the uptake represents inflammatory reaction, it is not an active disease process. Medical history and examination of the patient are essential to differentiate an active disease process from iatrogenic wound or physiologic reactions on a Ga 67 scan.

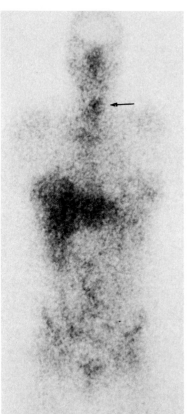
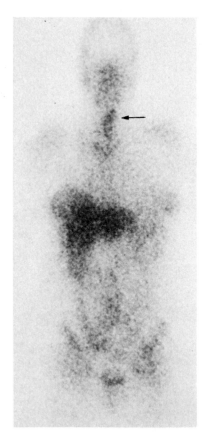

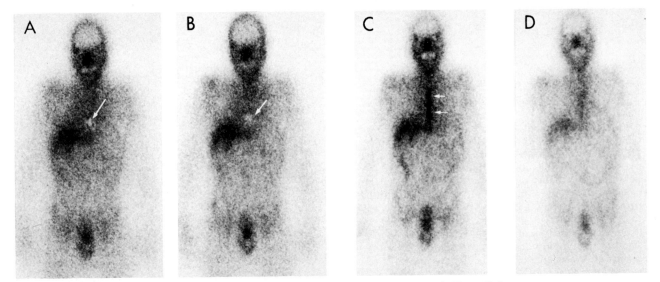

Case 11–19.—Pacemaker Artifact on Gallium Citrate Ga 67 Scan in Patient with Heart Failure

A and B, selective anterior planes of tomographic body gallium citrate Ga 67 scan on a 60-year-old man with myocardial disease show a round photon-deficient area in the midline anterior chest (arrow). The patient had a cardiac pacemaker implanted in the chest wall corresponding to the cold spot. In addition, prominent photon attenuation by the denture caused "open-mouth" appearance.

C, anterior plane Ga 67 scan on the same patient taken two weeks after a coronary artery bypass graft operation shows abnormal linear uptake in the sternum representing the thoracotomy scar. If the history of the recent thoracotomy had not been available, the finding would have indicated possible infection of the sternum.

D, follow-up scan obtained eight months after the cardiac surgery shows complete resolution of the Ga 67 uptake in the thoracotomy scar in the sternum.

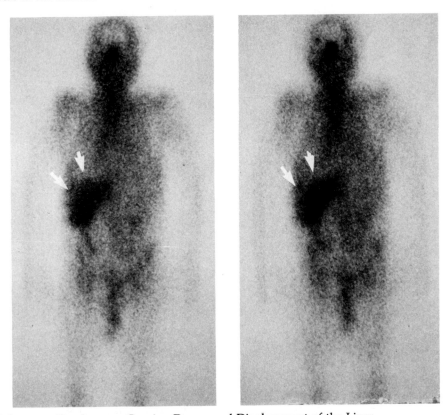

Case 11–20.—Pulmonary Emphysema Causing Downward Displacement of the Liver

Selective anterior planes of tomographic body gallium citrate Ga 67 scan show severely deformed and inferiorly displaced liver (arrows). The liver mimics a large Ga 67 positive mass lesion in the right upper abdomen. The patient, 65-year-old man, had a long history of heavy smoking and severe pulmonary emphysema, causing such severe downward displacement of the liver.

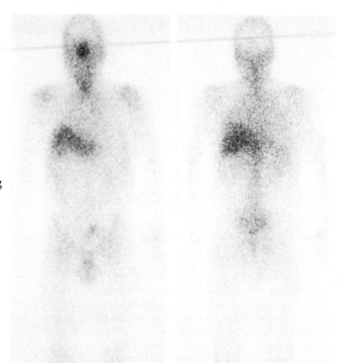

Case 11–21.—Elevated Right Diaphragm; High Position of the Liver

Whole body gallium citrate Ga 67 scan on a 50-year-old man, anterior **(left)** and posterior **(right)** sections of tomograms, shows abnormally high position of the liver, which appears as if it is in the thorax. The patient had a history of right pneumonectomy for lung carcinoma. Lack of gallium citrate Ga 67 uptake in the upper thoracic spine indicates prior radiation therapy to the chest.

Such high position of the liver may be seen in patients with ascites or paralyzed right diaphragm. However, the degree of the displacement is most prominent in cases of right pneumonectomy.

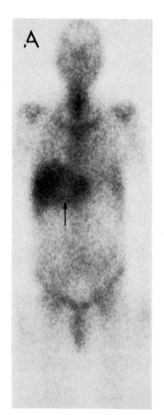
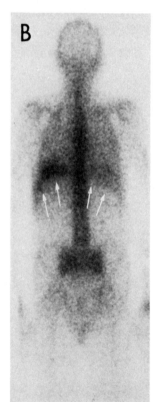
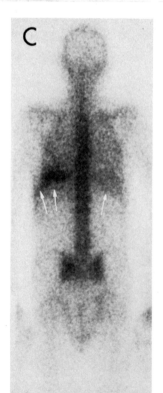
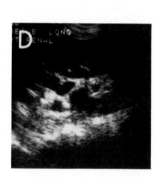
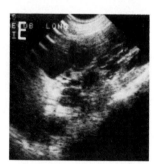

Case 11–22.—Empty Retroperitoneal Region Due to Polycystic Kidneys Demonstrated on a Gallium Citrate Ga 67 Scan

Selective anterior plane **(A)** and posterior planes **(B** and **C)** of tomographic gallium citrate Ga 67 scan obtained on a 71-year-old man show unusually prominent portahepatis **(A,** *arrow*), upward displacement of the posterior liver and spleen **(B** and **C)**, and clear (empty) retroperitoneal space. The posterior planes show no evidence of renal activity.

The patient had a long history of bilateral polycystic kidneys.

Ultrasonograms of the right **(D)** and left **(E)** kidneys confirmed very large, bilateral polycystic kidneys that caused the empty retroperitoneal space and prominent portahepatis (compression defect).

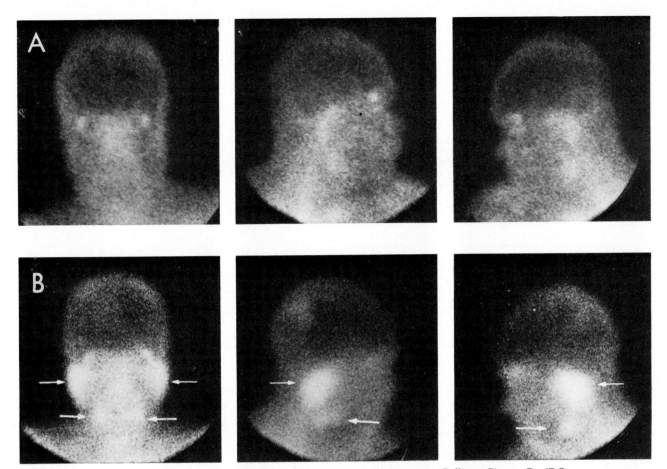

Case 11–23.—Increased Salivary Gland Uptake Secondary to Irradiation on a Gallium Citrate Ga 67 Scan

A, camera images of head and neck, anterior and both lateral views, obtained 48 hours after an intravenous injection of gallium citrate Ga 67 show normal distribution of the radionuclide in the lacrimal glands, in the nasopharynx, and salivary glands.

B, camera images of the head and neck Ga 67 scan, obtained 48 hours after the injection on a patient who underwent radiation therapy to the brain for a metastatic lung carcinoma, show intense activity in the parotid glands and also increased uptake in the submandibular glands *(arrows);* a frequent finding on a Ga 67 scan, postradiation sialitis.

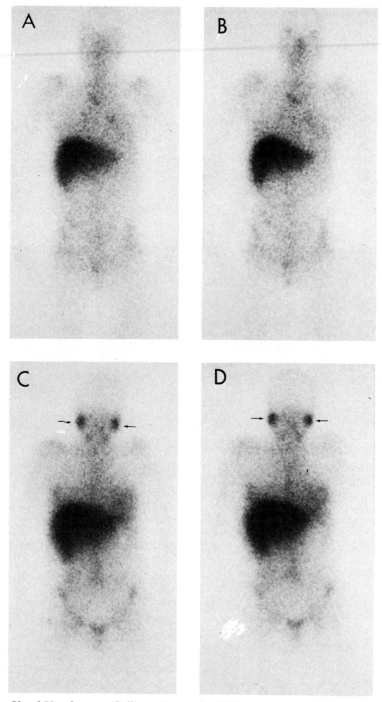

Case 11–24.—Salivary Gland Uptake on a Gallium Citrate Ga 67 Scan

A and **B**, selective anterior planes of tomographic gallium citrate Ga 67 scan obtained on a 43-year-old woman with carcinoma of the lung show areas of abnormal uptake in the lung and hilar region, but show normal uptake by the salivary glands. The scans also show normal Ga 67 uptake by a normal liver.

C and **D**, repeated Ga 67 scan on the same patient obtained two weeks after radiation therapy given to the chest. There is markedly increased uptake by the parotid glands *(arrows)*. Such Ga 67 uptake by the salivary gland due to radiation-induced sialitis is considered nonpathological. Increased uptake by the breast on the second scan indicates that the patient resumed taking birth control pill medications.

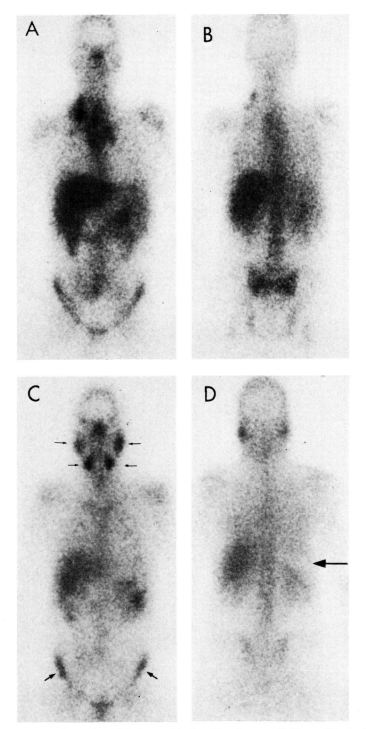

Case 11–25.—Radiation Sialitis of Parotid and Submandibular Glands on a Gallium Citrate Ga 67 Scan

A and **B,** selective anterior and posterior planes of a tomographic gallium citrate Ga 67 scan obtained on a 28-year-old man with extensive Hodgkin's lymphoma show multiple areas of abnormal uptake in the cervical and mediastinal nodes. But salivary glands were not visualized, a normal variant.

C and **D,** follow-up Ga 67 scan obtained on the same patient after radiation therapy to the neck and chest, bone marrow biopsy from the bilateral iliac crest, and splenectomy shows increased uptake by the parotid and submandibular glands (**C,** *arrows*), focal uptake in the anterior iliac crest (**C,** *arrows*), and a photon-deficient area representing the empty splenic bed (**D,** *arrow*).

Case 11–26.—Nonvisualization of the Spine on a Gallium Citrate Ga 67 Scan

Selective posterior planes of tomographic gallium citrate Ga 67 scan obtained on a 50-year-old man with Hodgkin's lymphoma show nonvisualization of the thoracic spine. The patient received irradiation therapy over the mediastinum for the lymphoma.

Such diminished Ga 67 uptake by the skeletal structure is mainly due to suppression of the bone marrow function by the radiation. Such radiation effects are seldom demonstrated on a bone scan with technetium Tc-99m phosphate compounds, unless the radiation dose reaches unusually high levels.

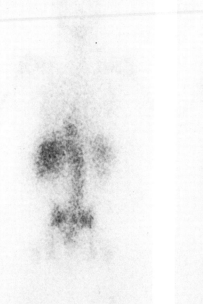
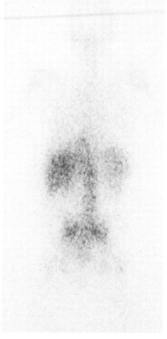

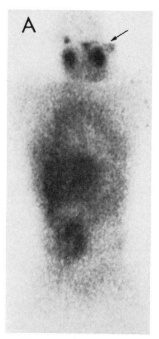
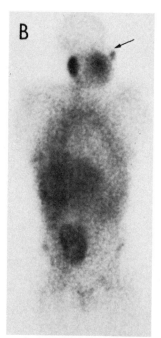
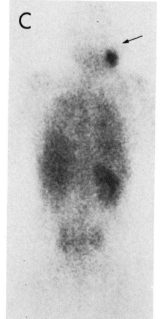
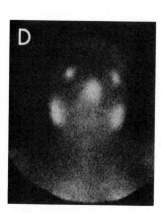

Case 11–27.—Motion Artifact on a Gallium Citrate Ga 67 Scan

Selective anterior planes (**A** and **B**) and posterior plane (**C**) of a tomographic gallium citrate Ga 67 scan obtained on a 35-year-old woman with extensive sarcoidosis show two large Ga 67 positive areas (?) in the neck *(arrow)*. The architecture of the skull is deformed. A repeated anterior camera image of the skull (**D**) shows increased uptake by the bilateral parotid gland without cervical mass lesion. The patient moved her head while the tomographic detectors were scanning the nasopharyngeal region. Because of the movement, there is obvious distortion of the anatomy, which may cause false interpretation of probable cervical mass lesions.

The patient had bilateral renal involvement, causing intense uptake. The right kidney is imaged in the anterior pelvis.

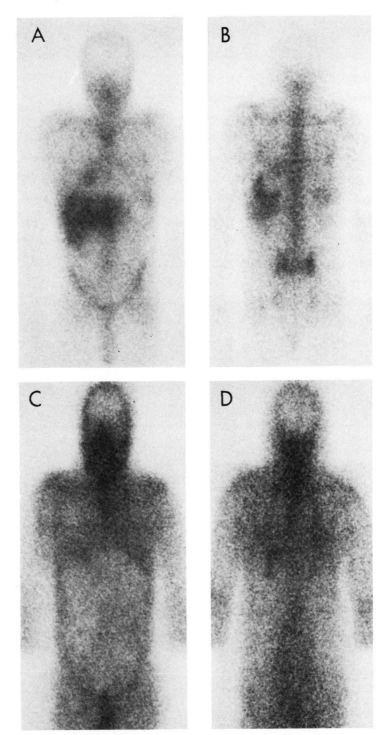

Case 11–28.—Effect of Chemotherapeutic Agents on Gallium Citrate Ga 67 Scan

A and **B,** selective anterior and posterior planes of a tomographic gallium citrate Ga 67 scan obtained on a 69-year-old man with lung carcinomas show abnormal uptake in the right lower lobe and the right hilar nodes. There is normal uptake by the liver and bones.

C and **D,** repeated scan obtained on the same patient shows nonvisualization of the liver and poor visualization of the carcinomas and bones. The patient received a dose of chemotherapeutic agents a few hours before the intravenous injection of Ga 67.

The second scan also shows elongated figure, which is an instrumental artifact, a minor malfunction of an electrical circuit board.

Comments: the mechanism for the blocking of Ga 67 uptake by the liver and tumors is not elucidated. A plausible cause of such a phenomenon is saturation of the Ga 67 binding site by the chemotherapeutic agents (Bekerman C., Pavel D.G., Bitran J., et al.: The effects of inadvertent administration of antineoplastic agents prior to Ga 67 injection: Concise communication. *J. Nucl. Med.* 25:430, 1984).

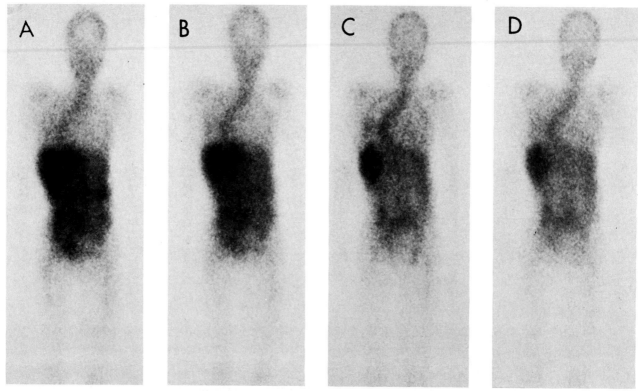

Case 11–29.—Effect of Severe Scoliosis of the Thoracic Spine on a Gallium Citrate Ga 67 Scan

Selective anterior (**A** and **B**) and posterior (**C** and **D**) planes of tomographic whole body gallium citrate Ga 67 scan obtained on a 53-year-old woman show a severe scoliosis of the thoracic spine. The scoliosis is causing increased uptake in the right lower lung due to compressed lung tissue. Similarly, displaced tissue of the right posterior liver is causing "hot" posterior liver, artifactitious Ga 67 positive findings.

Case 11–30.—Surgical Wound on a Gallium Citrate Ga 67 Scan

Selective anterior planes of a tomographic gallium citrate Ga 67 scan obtained on a 48-year-old man who had undergone a cholecystectomy four days earlier show a linear area of intense uptake in the right upper abdomen *(arrows)*.

In addition, normal excretion of the Ga 67 in the transverse, splenic flexure, and descending colon is noted.

The linear intense uptake represented the transverse surgical incision wound in the abdominal wall.

Such Ga 67 uptake in a surgical wound may be seen for as long as two months after a major surgery.

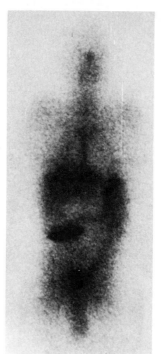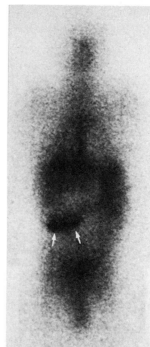

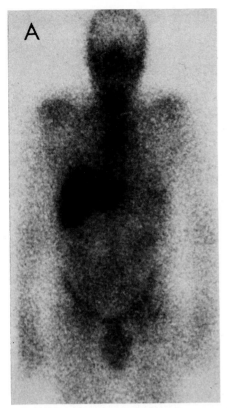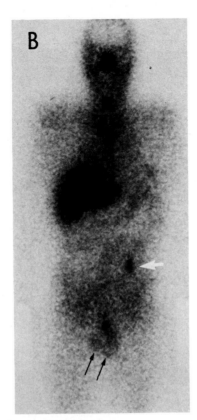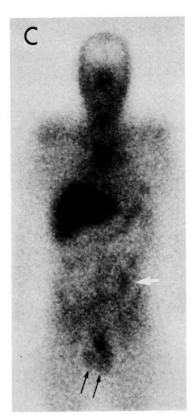

Case 11–31.—Surgical Wound on a Gallium Citrate Ga 67 Scan

A, selective anterior plane of tomographic gallium citrate Ga 67 scan obtained on a 73-year-old man with colon carcinoma shows normal distribution of the radionuclide.

B and **C,** follow-up scan, anterior planes, obtained 16 months after surgical resection of colon carcinoma, shows an abnormal focal uptake in the left lower abdomen *(white arrow)*. This focal Ga 67 concentration represented the colostomy site. Such Ga 67 positive surgical wound should not be misinterpreted as focus of infection or a tumor. Unusually prominent testicular uptake *(black arrows)* is occasionally seen in patients without pathological process in the testes.

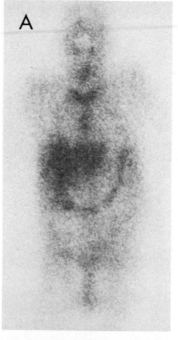
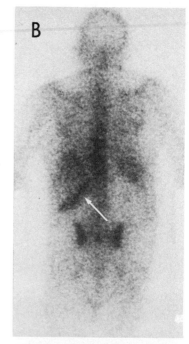

Case 11–32.—Retroperitoneal Displacement of the Colon Mimics Gallium Citrate Ga 67-Positive Lesion

Selective anterior **(A)** and posterior **(B)** planes of a tomographic gallium citrate Ga 67 scan obtained on a 70-year-old man with a history of renal carcinoma. The posterior plane shows a linear activity in the right retroperitoneal region *(arrow)*.

Right lateral **(C)** and posterior **(D)** camera images reveal that there is a marked displacement of the hepatic flexure of the colon into the right renal impression *(arrows)*.

This patient had undergone right nephrectomy nine years earlier that led the shift of position of the colon posteriorly.

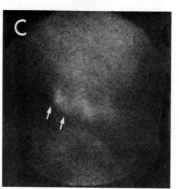
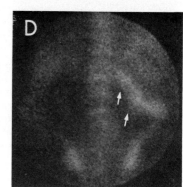

Case 11–33.—Intense Breast Activity on a Gallium Citrate Ga 67 Scan Due to Birth Control Pills

Selective anterior planes of whole body tomographic gallium citrate Ga 67 scan on a 23-year-old woman show symmetrical, intense uptake in the breast. The patient was taking daily birth control pills that had been documented to cause Ga 67 uptake in the breast, especially prominent in young women (Bekerman C., Hoffer P.B., Bitran J.D., et al.: Gallium-67 citrate imaging studies of the lung. *Semin. Nucl. Med.* 10:286, 1980).

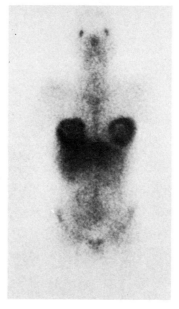
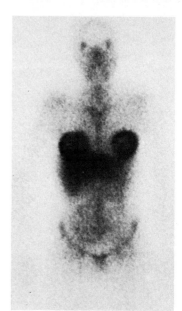

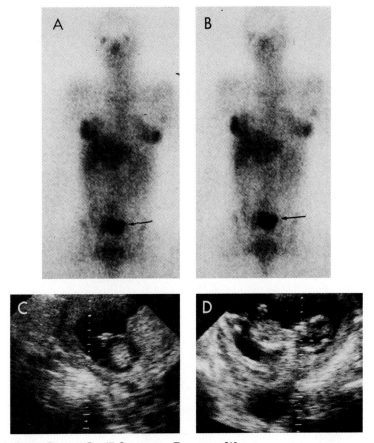

Case 11–34.—Normal Gallium Citrate Ga 67 Scan on a Pregnant Woman

Selective anterior planes of tomographic gallium citrate Ga 67 scan (**A** and **B**) obtained on a 32-year-old woman with Hodgkin's lymphoma show intense activity in the breast and in the uterus (*arrow*).

The patient was unaware of her pregnancy at the time of admission. During the staging work-up, computerized tomography of the pelvis revealed her pregnancy. The ultrasonograms (**C** and **D**) revealed the fetus of 12 weeks' gestation.

The Ga 67 scan was performed after the patient and her physician decided to abort the fetus and start chemotherapy for her lymphomas.

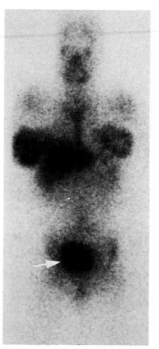
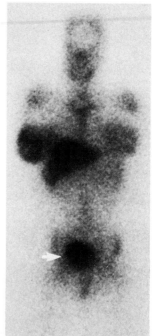

Case 11–35.—Intense Activity in the Breast and the Postpartum Uterus on a Gallium Citrate Ga 67 Scan

Selective anterior planes of tomographic gallium citrate Ga 67 scan obtained on a 23-year-old woman two days after a parturition show intense Ga 67 uptake by the breast and by the uterus *(arrow)*.

The scan was taken immediately after the urinary bladder was emptied. Initially, the patient had fever, and possible pelvic abscess was suspected; however, no abscess was found in the pelvis. The intense localization of Ga 67 was due to severe injury of the postpartum uterus.

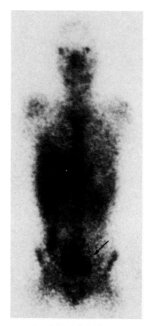
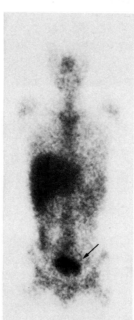
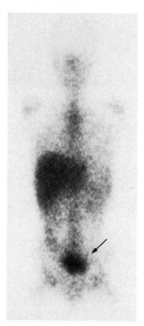

Case 11–36.—Demonstration of a Gestating Uterus on a Gallium Citrate Ga 67 Scan; Example Case

Selective anterior slices of tomographic gallium citrate Ga 67 body scan obtained 72 hours after an intravenous dose of 10 mCi on a 32-year-old woman with right lung carcinoma show an area of intense Ga 67 uptake in the pelvis *(arrows)*.

The patient denied any knowledge of her pregnancy; however, it was later documented that she was 20 weeks pregnant, and no other mass was found in the pelvis by ultrasonography.

Comments: precise localization of Ga 67 in a gestating uterus has not been documented. An earlier report described that the location of the Ga 67 uptake corresponded to the placenta (Newman R.A., Gallagher J.G., Clements J.P., et al.: Demonstration of Ga 67 localization in human placenta. *J. Nucl. Med.* 19:504, 1978). In the case shown here Ga 67 appears to be localized more in the anterior wall of the uterus, suggesting it probably represents uptake by the placenta.

The patient decided to carry her pregnancy; therefore, radiation dose to the fetus became a matter of concern.

Radiation dose from a 10-mCi dose of Ga 67 to the colon is 9 rad, and to the kidney is 5 rad (MIRD Committee: Dose estimate report No. 2. Summary of current radiation dose estimates to humans from 66Ga-, 67Ga-, 68Ga-, and 72Ga-Citrate. *J. Nucl. Med.* 14:755, 1973.) Lack of basic data does not allow one to make accurate estimates of the radiation dose to the fetus. However, total radiation absorbed dose to the 20-week-gestational fetus from a 10-mCi dose of ^{67}Ga can be estimated as 9–30 rad.

(Courtesy of William B. Martin, M.D., Department of Radiology, Division of Nuclear Medicine, The University of Chicago Hospital, Chicago.)

Index